H&P Notebook

Medical Creations

LIST OF ABBREVIATIONS

BL	-	Bilateral
BMI	-	Body mass index
BP	-	Blood pressure
CAD	-	Coronary artery disease
CN	-	Cranial nerve
CTAB	-	Clear to auscultation bilaterally
CV	-	Cardiovascular
CVA	-	Cerebrovascular accident
CXR	-	Chest X-ray
DOA	-	Date of admission
DM	-	Diabetes mellitus
EKG	-	Electrocardiography
Endo	-	Endocrine
ENT	-	Ear nose throat
EOMI	-	Extra ocular movements intact
GI	-	Gastrointestinal
GU	-	Genitourinary
HEENT	-	Head, eyes, ears, nose and throat
HTN	-	Hypertension
JVD	-	Jugular venous distention
LAD	-	Lymphadenopathy
MMM	-	Mucous membranes moist
m/r/g	-	Murmurs/rubs/gallops
MSK	-	Musculoskeletal
NC/AT	-	Normocephalic, atraumatic
ND/NT	-	Non-distended/non-tender
Neuro	-	Neurologic
PERRL	-	Pupils equal, round and reactive to light
Psych	-	Psychiatric
Resp	-	Respiratory
ROM	-	Range of motion
ROS	-	Review of systems
RR	-	Respiratory rate
RRR	-	Regular rate and rhythm
r/r/w	-	rales/rhonchi/wheezes
S1/S2	-	First and second heart sounds
SaO_2	-	Oxygen saturation
Temp	-	Temperature
TM	-	Tympanic membrane
WNL	-	Within normal limits

Date:	Patient Name:	Age:	Gender:
DOA:	Room #:	Bed:	

Chief Complaint:

History of Present Illness:

Past Medical History: (HTN/DM/CAD/CVA)

Medications:

Past Surgical History:

Family History:

Social History:

Occupation: Lives with: Relationship:

Drug/substance abuse history if any: (alcohol/tobacco/drugs)

Allergies:

Review of Systems: (Describe if not WNL)

General	☐ WNL / ☐ Other	**GI**	☐ WNL / ☐ Other
Skin	☐ WNL / ☐ Other	**GU**	☐ WNL / ☐ Other
ENT	☐ WNL / ☐ Other	**MSK**	☐ WNL / ☐ Other
Eyes	☐ WNL / ☐ Other	**Neuro**	☐ WNL / ☐ Other
CV	☐ WNL / ☐ Other	**Endo**	☐ WNL / ☐ Other
Resp	☐ WNL / ☐ Other	**Psych**	☐ WNL / ☐ Other

ROS additional notes

Physical Exam:

Vitals: Pulse: BP: RR: Temp:
SaO$_2$: Height: Weight: BMI:

General	(NAD, alert, interactive)
HEENT	(NC/AT, MMM, PERRL, EOMI, BL TM intact and reactive to light, BL sclera anicteric)
Neck	(supple, no LAD, no JVD, no thyromegaly)
Cardiovascular	(RRR, S1/S2 normal, no m/r/g)
Respiratory	(CTAB, no r/r/w)
Abdominal	(soft, ND/NT, no masses, normal bowel sounds)
Neurologic	(no focal deficit, CN II-XII intact)
Extremities	(normal tone and ROM)
Skin	(intact, no rashes/lesions/erythema)

Physical exam additional notes:

Labs:

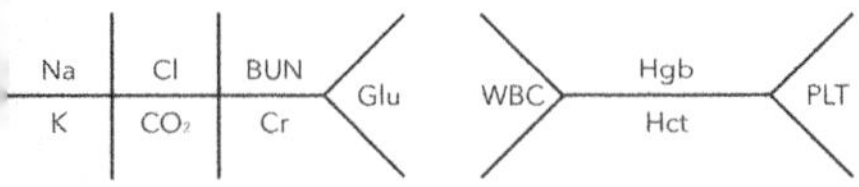

Other Labs:

Studies: (EKG, CXR, other imaging studies)

Impression / Assessment:

Differential Diagnosis:

Plan:

Updates / Notes:

To Do:

Date: Patient Name: Age: Gender:

DOA: Room #: Bed:

Chief Complaint:

History of Present Illness:

Past Medical History: (HTN/DM/CAD/CVA)

Medications:

Past Surgical History:

Family History:

Social History:

Occupation: Lives with: Relationship:

Drug/substance abuse history if any: (alcohol/tobacco/drugs)

Allergies:

Review of Systems: (Describe if not WNL)

General	☐ WNL / ☐ Other	**GI**	☐ WNL / ☐ Other
Skin	☐ WNL / ☐ Other	**GU**	☐ WNL / ☐ Other
ENT	☐ WNL / ☐ Other	**MSK**	☐ WNL / ☐ Other
Eyes	☐ WNL / ☐ Other	**Neuro**	☐ WNL / ☐ Other
CV	☐ WNL / ☐ Other	**Endo**	☐ WNL / ☐ Other
Resp	☐ WNL / ☐ Other	**Psych**	☐ WNL / ☐ Other

ROS additional notes

Physical Exam:

Vitals:	Pulse:	BP:	RR:	Temp:
	SaO_2:	Height:	Weight:	BMI:

General	(NAD, alert, interactive)
HEENT	(NC/AT, MMM, PERRL, EOMI, BL TM intact and reactive to light, BL sclera anicteric)
Neck	(supple, no LAD, no JVD, no thyromegaly)
Cardiovascular	(RRR, S1/S2 normal, no m/r/g)
Respiratory	(CTAB, no r/r/w)
Abdominal	(soft, ND/NT, no masses, normal bowel sounds)
Neurologic	(no focal deficit, CN II-XII intact)
Extremities	(normal tone and ROM)
Skin	(intact, no rashes/lesions/erythema)

Physical exam additional notes:

Labs:

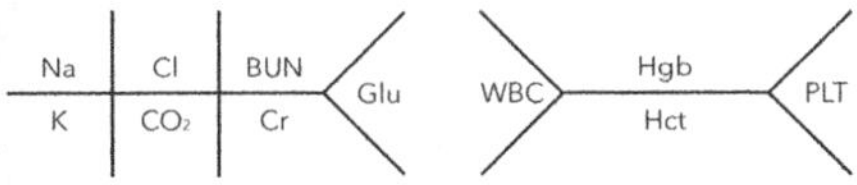

Other Labs:

Studies: (EKG, CXR, other imaging studies)

Impression / Assessment:

Differential Diagnosis:

Plan:

Updates / Notes:

To Do:

Patient Name: Age: Gender:

Room #: Bed:

omplaint:

History of Present Illness:

Past Medical History: (HTN/DM/CAD/CVA)

Medications:

Past Surgical History:

Family History:

Social History:

Occupation: Lives with: Relationship:

Drug/substance abuse history if any: (alcohol/tobacco/drugs)

Allergies:

Review of Systems: (Describe if not WNL)

General	☐ WNL / ☐ Other	**GI**	☐ WNL / ☐ Other
Skin	☐ WNL / ☐ Other	**GU**	☐ WNL / ☐ Other
ENT	☐ WNL / ☐ Other	**MSK**	☐ WNL / ☐ Other
Eyes	☐ WNL / ☐ Other	**Neuro**	☐ WNL / ☐ Other
CV	☐ WNL / ☐ Other	**Endo**	☐ WNL / ☐ Other
Resp	☐ WNL / ☐ Other	**Psych**	☐ WNL / ☐ Other

ROS additional notes

Physical Exam:

Vitals:	Pulse:	BP:	RR:	Temp:
	SaO_2:	Height:	Weight:	BMI:

General	(NAD, alert, interactive)
HEENT	(NC/AT, MMM, PERRL, EOMI, BL TM intact and reactive to light, BL sclera anicteric)
Neck	(supple, no LAD, no JVD, no thyromegaly)
Cardiovascular	(RRR, S1/S2 normal, no m/r/g)
Respiratory	(CTAB, no r/r/w)
Abdominal	(soft, ND/NT, no masses, normal bowel sounds)
Neurologic	(no focal deficit, CN II-XII intact)
Extremities	(normal tone and ROM)
Skin	(intact, no rashes/lesions/erythema)

Physical exam additional notes:

Labs:

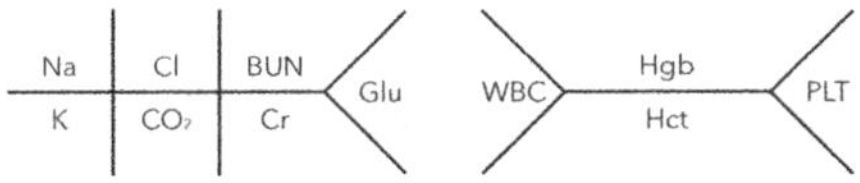

Other Labs:

Studies: (EKG, CXR, other imaging studies)

Impression / Assessment:

Differential Diagnosis:

Plan:

Updates / Notes:

To Do:

Date: Patient Name: Age: Gender:

DOA: Room #: Bed:

Chief Complaint:

History of Present Illness:

Past Medical History: (HTN/DM/CAD/CVA)

Medications:

Past Surgical History:

Family History:

Social History:

Occupation: Lives with: Relationship:

Drug/substance abuse history if any: (alcohol/tobacco/drugs)

Allergies:

Review of Systems: (Describe if not WNL)

General	☐ WNL / ☐ Other	**GI**	☐ WNL / ☐ Other
Skin	☐ WNL / ☐ Other	**GU**	☐ WNL / ☐ Other
ENT	☐ WNL / ☐ Other	**MSK**	☐ WNL / ☐ Other
Eyes	☐ WNL / ☐ Other	**Neuro**	☐ WNL / ☐ Other
CV	☐ WNL / ☐ Other	**Endo**	☐ WNL / ☐ Other
Resp	☐ WNL / ☐ Other	**Psych**	☐ WNL / ☐ Other

ROS additional notes

Physical Exam:

Vitals: Pulse: BP: RR: Temp:
SaO$_2$: Height: Weight: BMI:

General	(NAD, alert, interactive)
HEENT	(NC/AT, MMM, PERRL, EOMI, BL TM intact and reactive to light, BL sclera anicteric)
Neck	(supple, no LAD, no JVD, no thyromegaly)
Cardiovascular	(RRR, S1/S2 normal, no m/r/g)
Respiratory	(CTAB, no r/r/w)
Abdominal	(soft, ND/NT, no masses, normal bowel sounds)
Neurologic	(no focal deficit, CN II-XII intact)
Extremities	(normal tone and ROM)
Skin	(intact, no rashes/lesions/erythema)

Physical exam additional notes:

Labs:

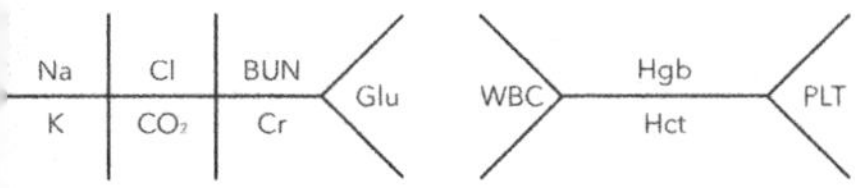

Other Labs:

Studies: (EKG, CXR, other imaging studies)

Impression / Assessment:

Differential Diagnosis:

Plan:

Updates / Notes:

To Do:

Date: Patient Name: Age: Gender:

DOA: Room #: Bed:

Chief Complaint:

History of Present Illness:

Past Medical History: (HTN/DM/CAD/CVA)

Medications:

Past Surgical History:

Family History:

Social History:

Occupation: Lives with: Relationship:

Drug/substance abuse history if any: (alcohol/tobacco/drugs)

Allergies:

Review of Systems: (Describe if not WNL)

General	☐ WNL / ☐ Other	**GI**	☐ WNL / ☐ Other
Skin	☐ WNL / ☐ Other	**GU**	☐ WNL / ☐ Other
ENT	☐ WNL / ☐ Other	**MSK**	☐ WNL / ☐ Other
Eyes	☐ WNL / ☐ Other	**Neuro**	☐ WNL / ☐ Other
CV	☐ WNL / ☐ Other	**Endo**	☐ WNL / ☐ Other
Resp	☐ WNL / ☐ Other	**Psych**	☐ WNL / ☐ Other

ROS additional notes

Physical Exam:

Vitals: Pulse: BP: RR: Temp:
SaO_2: Height: Weight: BMI:

General	(NAD, alert, interactive)
HEENT	(NC/AT, MMM, PERRL, EOMI, BL TM intact and reactive to light, BL sclera anicteric)
Neck	(supple, no LAD, no JVD, no thyromegaly)
Cardiovascular	(RRR, S1/S2 normal, no m/r/g)
Respiratory	(CTAB, no r/r/w)
Abdominal	(soft, ND/NT, no masses, normal bowel sounds)
Neurologic	(no focal deficit, CN II-XII intact)
Extremities	(normal tone and ROM)
Skin	(intact, no rashes/lesions/erythema)

Physical exam additional notes:

Labs:

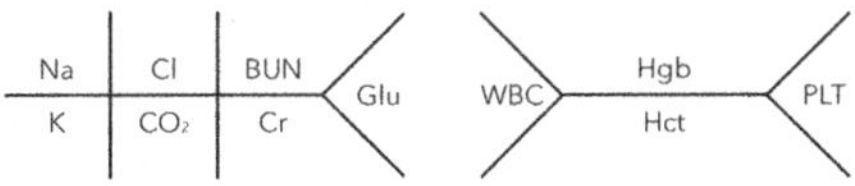

Other Labs:

Studies: (EKG, CXR, other imaging studies)

Impression / Assessment:

Differential Diagnosis:

Plan:

Updates / Notes:

To Do:

Date:	Patient Name:		Age:	Gender:
DOA:	Room #:	Bed:		

Chief Complaint:

History of Present Illness:

Past Medical History: (HTN/DM/CAD/CVA)

Medications:

Past Surgical History:	**Family History:**

Social History:

Occupation: Lives with: Relationship:

Drug/substance abuse history if any: (alcohol/tobacco/drugs)

Allergies:

Review of Systems: (Describe if not WNL)

General	☐ WNL / ☐ Other	**GI**	☐ WNL / ☐ Other
Skin	☐ WNL / ☐ Other	**GU**	☐ WNL / ☐ Other
ENT	☐ WNL / ☐ Other	**MSK**	☐ WNL / ☐ Other
Eyes	☐ WNL / ☐ Other	**Neuro**	☐ WNL / ☐ Other
CV	☐ WNL / ☐ Other	**Endo**	☐ WNL / ☐ Other
Resp	☐ WNL / ☐ Other	**Psych**	☐ WNL / ☐ Other

ROS additional notes

Physical Exam:

Vitals: Pulse: BP: RR: Temp:
SaO$_2$: Height: Weight: BMI:

General	(NAD, alert, interactive)
HEENT	(NC/AT, MMM, PERRL, EOMI, BL TM intact and reactive to light, BL sclera anicteric)
Neck	(supple, no LAD, no JVD, no thyromegaly)
Cardiovascular	(RRR, S1/S2 normal, no m/r/g)
Respiratory	(CTAB, no r/r/w)
Abdominal	(soft, ND/NT, no masses, normal bowel sounds)
Neurologic	(no focal deficit, CN II-XII intact)
Extremities	(normal tone and ROM)
Skin	(intact, no rashes/lesions/erythema)

Physical exam additional notes:

Labs:

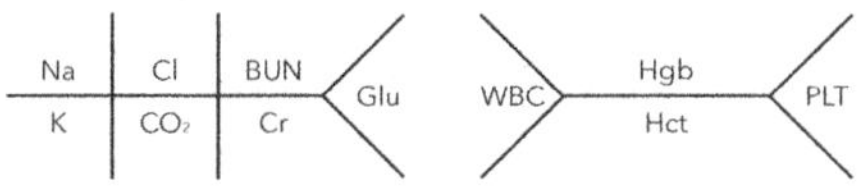

Other Labs:

Studies: (EKG, CXR, other imaging studies)

Impression / Assessment:

Differential Diagnosis:

Plan:

Updates / Notes:

To Do:

Date: Patient Name: Age: Gender:

DOA: Room #: Bed:

Chief Complaint:

History of Present Illness:

Past Medical History: (HTN/DM/CAD/CVA)

Medications:

Past Surgical History:

Family History:

Social History:

Occupation: Lives with: Relationship:

Drug/substance abuse history if any: (alcohol/tobacco/drugs)

Allergies:

Review of Systems: (Describe if not WNL)

General	☐ WNL / ☐ Other	**GI**	☐ WNL / ☐ Other
Skin	☐ WNL / ☐ Other	**GU**	☐ WNL / ☐ Other
ENT	☐ WNL / ☐ Other	**MSK**	☐ WNL / ☐ Other
Eyes	☐ WNL / ☐ Other	**Neuro**	☐ WNL / ☐ Other
CV	☐ WNL / ☐ Other	**Endo**	☐ WNL / ☐ Other
Resp	☐ WNL / ☐ Other	**Psych**	☐ WNL / ☐ Other

ROS additional notes

Physical Exam:

Vitals: Pulse: BP: RR: Temp:
SaO$_2$: Height: Weight: BMI:

General	(NAD, alert, interactive)
HEENT	(NC/AT, MMM, PERRL, EOMI, BL TM intact and reactive to light, BL sclera anicteric)
Neck	(supple, no LAD, no JVD, no thyromegaly)
Cardiovascular	(RRR, S1/S2 normal, no m/r/g)
Respiratory	(CTAB, no r/r/w)
Abdominal	(soft, ND/NT, no masses, normal bowel sounds)
Neurologic	(no focal deficit, CN II-XII intact)
Extremities	(normal tone and ROM)
Skin	(intact, no rashes/lesions/erythema)

Physical exam additional notes:

Labs:

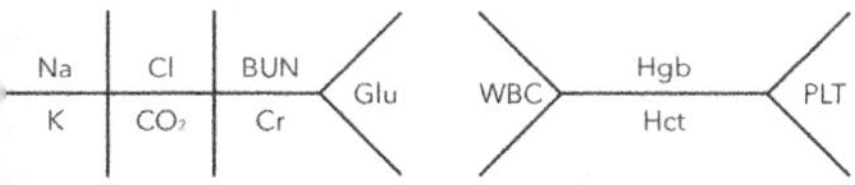

Other Labs:

Studies: (EKG, CXR, other imaging studies)

Impression / Assessment:

Differential Diagnosis:

Plan:

Updates / Notes:

To Do:

Date: Patient Name: Age: Gender:

DOA: Room #: Bed:

Chief Complaint:

History of Present Illness:

Past Medical History: (HTN/DM/CAD/CVA)

Medications:

Past Surgical History:

Family History:

Social History:

Occupation: Lives with: Relationship:

Drug/substance abuse history if any: (alcohol/tobacco/drugs)

Allergies:

Review of Systems: (Describe if not WNL)

General	☐ WNL / ☐ Other	**GI**	☐ WNL / ☐ Other
Skin	☐ WNL / ☐ Other	**GU**	☐ WNL / ☐ Other
ENT	☐ WNL / ☐ Other	**MSK**	☐ WNL / ☐ Other
Eyes	☐ WNL / ☐ Other	**Neuro**	☐ WNL / ☐ Other
CV	☐ WNL / ☐ Other	**Endo**	☐ WNL / ☐ Other
Resp	☐ WNL / ☐ Other	**Psych**	☐ WNL / ☐ Other

ROS additional notes

Physical Exam:

Vitals: Pulse: BP: RR: Temp:
SaO$_2$: Height: Weight: BMI:

General	(NAD, alert, interactive)
HEENT	(NC/AT, MMM, PERRL, EOMI, BL TM intact and reactive to light, BL sclera anicteric)
Neck	(supple, no LAD, no JVD, no thyromegaly)
Cardiovascular	(RRR, S1/S2 normal, no m/r/g)
Respiratory	(CTAB, no r/r/w)
Abdominal	(soft, ND/NT, no masses, normal bowel sounds)
Neurologic	(no focal deficit, CN II-XII intact)
Extremities	(normal tone and ROM)
Skin	(intact, no rashes/lesions/erythema)

Physical exam additional notes:

Labs:

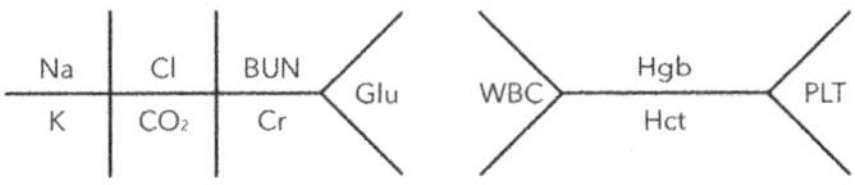

Other Labs:

Studies: (EKG, CXR, other imaging studies)

Impression / Assessment:

Differential Diagnosis:

Plan:

Updates / Notes:

To Do:

Date: Patient Name: Age: Gender:

DOA: Room #: Bed:

Chief Complaint:

History of Present Illness:

Past Medical History: (HTN/DM/CAD/CVA)

Medications:

Past Surgical History:

Family History:

Social History:

Occupation: Lives with: Relationship:

Drug/substance abuse history if any: (alcohol/tobacco/drugs)

Allergies:

Review of Systems: (Describe if not WNL)

General	☐ WNL / ☐ Other	**GI**	☐ WNL / ☐ Other
Skin	☐ WNL / ☐ Other	**GU**	☐ WNL / ☐ Other
ENT	☐ WNL / ☐ Other	**MSK**	☐ WNL / ☐ Other
Eyes	☐ WNL / ☐ Other	**Neuro**	☐ WNL / ☐ Other
CV	☐ WNL / ☐ Other	**Endo**	☐ WNL / ☐ Other
Resp	☐ WNL / ☐ Other	**Psych**	☐ WNL / ☐ Other

ROS additional notes

Physical Exam:

Vitals:	Pulse:	BP:	RR:	Temp:
	SaO_2:	Height:	Weight:	BMI:

General	(NAD, alert, interactive)
HEENT	(NC/AT, MMM, PERRL, EOMI, BL TM intact and reactive to light, BL sclera anicteric)
Neck	(supple, no LAD, no JVD, no thyromegaly)
Cardiovascular	(RRR, S1/S2 normal, no m/r/g)
Respiratory	(CTAB, no r/r/w)
Abdominal	(soft, ND/NT, no masses, normal bowel sounds)
Neurologic	(no focal deficit, CN II-XII intact)
Extremities	(normal tone and ROM)
Skin	(intact, no rashes/lesions/erythema)

Physical exam additional notes:

Labs:

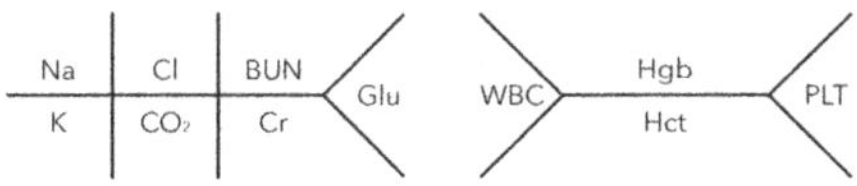

Other Labs:

Studies: (EKG, CXR, other imaging studies)

Impression / Assessment:

Differential Diagnosis:

Plan:

Updates / Notes:

To Do:

Date: Patient Name: Age: Gender:

DOA: Room #: Bed:

Chief Complaint:

History of Present Illness:

Past Medical History: (HTN/DM/CAD/CVA)

Medications:

Past Surgical History:

Family History:

Social History:

Occupation: Lives with: Relationship:

Drug/substance abuse history if any: (alcohol/tobacco/drugs)

Allergies:

Review of Systems: (Describe if not WNL)

General	☐ WNL / ☐ Other	**GI**	☐ WNL / ☐ Other
Skin	☐ WNL / ☐ Other	**GU**	☐ WNL / ☐ Other
ENT	☐ WNL / ☐ Other	**MSK**	☐ WNL / ☐ Other
Eyes	☐ WNL / ☐ Other	**Neuro**	☐ WNL / ☐ Other
CV	☐ WNL / ☐ Other	**Endo**	☐ WNL / ☐ Other
Resp	☐ WNL / ☐ Other	**Psych**	☐ WNL / ☐ Other

ROS additional notes

Physical Exam:

Vitals:	Pulse:	BP:	RR:	Temp:
	SaO_2:	Height:	Weight:	BMI:

General	(NAD, alert, interactive)
HEENT	(NC/AT, MMM, PERRL, EOMI, BL TM intact and reactive to light, BL sclera anicteric)
Neck	(supple, no LAD, no JVD, no thyromegaly)
Cardiovascular	(RRR, S1/S2 normal, no m/r/g)
Respiratory	(CTAB, no r/r/w)
Abdominal	(soft, ND/NT, no masses, normal bowel sounds)
Neurologic	(no focal deficit, CN II-XII intact)
Extremities	(normal tone and ROM)
Skin	(intact, no rashes/lesions/erythema)

Physical exam additional notes:

Labs:

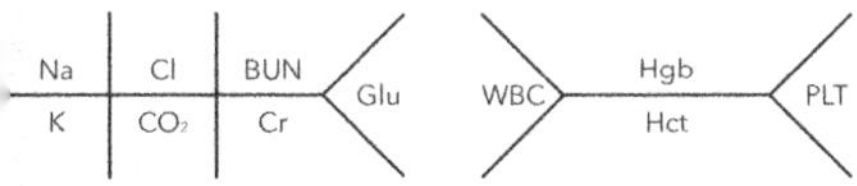

Other Labs:

Studies: (EKG, CXR, other imaging studies)

Impression / Assessment:

Differential Diagnosis:

Plan:

Updates / Notes:

To Do:

Date: Patient Name: Age: Gender:

DOA: Room #: Bed:

Chief Complaint:

History of Present Illness:

Past Medical History: (HTN/DM/CAD/CVA)

Medications:

Past Surgical History:

Family History:

Social History:

Occupation: Lives with: Relationship:

Drug/substance abuse history if any: (alcohol/tobacco/drugs)

Allergies:

Review of Systems: (Describe if not WNL)

General	☐ WNL / ☐ Other	**GI**	☐ WNL / ☐ Other
Skin	☐ WNL / ☐ Other	**GU**	☐ WNL / ☐ Other
ENT	☐ WNL / ☐ Other	**MSK**	☐ WNL / ☐ Other
Eyes	☐ WNL / ☐ Other	**Neuro**	☐ WNL / ☐ Other
CV	☐ WNL / ☐ Other	**Endo**	☐ WNL / ☐ Other
Resp	☐ WNL / ☐ Other	**Psych**	☐ WNL / ☐ Other

ROS additional notes

Physical Exam:

Vitals: Pulse: BP: RR: Temp:

SaO$_2$: Height: Weight: BMI:

General	(NAD, alert, interactive)
HEENT	(NC/AT, MMM, PERRL, EOMI, BL TM intact and reactive to light, BL sclera anicteric)
Neck	(supple, no LAD, no JVD, no thyromegaly)
Cardiovascular	(RRR, S1/S2 normal, no m/r/g)
Respiratory	(CTAB, no r/r/w)
Abdominal	(soft, ND/NT, no masses, normal bowel sounds)
Neurologic	(no focal deficit, CN II-XII intact)
Extremities	(normal tone and ROM)
Skin	(intact, no rashes/lesions/erythema)

Physical exam additional notes:

Labs:

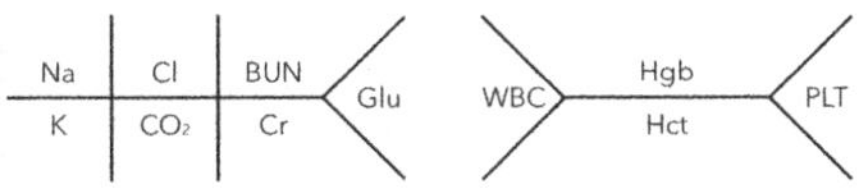

Other Labs:

Studies: (EKG, CXR, other imaging studies)

Impression / Assessment:

Differential Diagnosis:

Plan:

Updates / Notes:

To Do:

Date: Patient Name: Age: Gender:

DOA: Room #: Bed:

Chief Complaint:

History of Present Illness:

Past Medical History: (HTN/DM/CAD/CVA)

Medications:

Past Surgical History:

Family History:

Social History:

Occupation: Lives with: Relationship:

Drug/substance abuse history if any: (alcohol/tobacco/drugs)

Allergies:

Review of Systems: (Describe if not WNL)

General	☐ WNL / ☐ Other	**GI**	☐ WNL / ☐ Other
Skin	☐ WNL / ☐ Other	**GU**	☐ WNL / ☐ Other
ENT	☐ WNL / ☐ Other	**MSK**	☐ WNL / ☐ Other
Eyes	☐ WNL / ☐ Other	**Neuro**	☐ WNL / ☐ Other
CV	☐ WNL / ☐ Other	**Endo**	☐ WNL / ☐ Other
Resp	☐ WNL / ☐ Other	**Psych**	☐ WNL / ☐ Other

ROS additional notes

Physical Exam:

Vitals: Pulse: BP: RR: Temp:

SaO$_2$: Height: Weight: BMI:

General	(NAD, alert, interactive)
HEENT	(NC/AT, MMM, PERRL, EOMI, BL TM intact and reactive to light, BL sclera anicteric)
Neck	(supple, no LAD, no JVD, no thyromegaly)
Cardiovascular	(RRR, S1/S2 normal, no m/r/g)
Respiratory	(CTAB, no r/r/w)
Abdominal	(soft, ND/NT, no masses, normal bowel sounds)
Neurologic	(no focal deficit, CN II-XII intact)
Extremities	(normal tone and ROM)
Skin	(intact, no rashes/lesions/erythema)

Physical exam additional notes:

Labs:

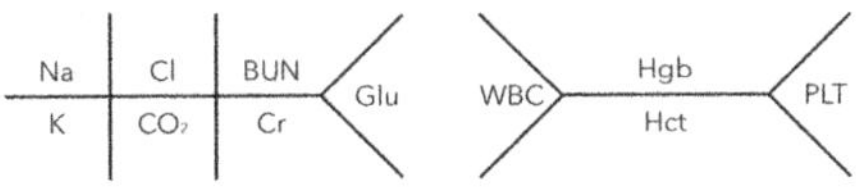

Other Labs:

Studies: (EKG, CXR, other imaging studies)

Impression / Assessment:

Differential Diagnosis:

Plan:

Updates / Notes:

To Do:

Date: Patient Name: Age: Gender:

DOA: Room #: Bed:

Chief Complaint:

History of Present Illness:

Past Medical History: (HTN/DM/CAD/CVA)

Medications:

Past Surgical History:

Family History:

Social History:

Occupation: Lives with: Relationship:

Drug/substance abuse history if any: (alcohol/tobacco/drugs)

Allergies:

Review of Systems: (Describe if not WNL)

General	☐ WNL / ☐ Other	**GI**	☐ WNL / ☐ Other
Skin	☐ WNL / ☐ Other	**GU**	☐ WNL / ☐ Other
ENT	☐ WNL / ☐ Other	**MSK**	☐ WNL / ☐ Other
Eyes	☐ WNL / ☐ Other	**Neuro**	☐ WNL / ☐ Other
CV	☐ WNL / ☐ Other	**Endo**	☐ WNL / ☐ Other
Resp	☐ WNL / ☐ Other	**Psych**	☐ WNL / ☐ Other

ROS additional notes

Physical Exam:

Vitals:	Pulse:	BP:	RR:	Temp:
	SaO_2:	Height:	Weight:	BMI:

General	(NAD, alert, interactive)
HEENT	(NC/AT, MMM, PERRL, EOMI, BL TM intact and reactive to light, BL sclera anicteric)
Neck	(supple, no LAD, no JVD, no thyromegaly)
Cardiovascular	(RRR, S1/S2 normal, no m/r/g)
Respiratory	(CTAB, no r/r/w)
Abdominal	(soft, ND/NT, no masses, normal bowel sounds)
Neurologic	(no focal deficit, CN II-XII intact)
Extremities	(normal tone and ROM)
Skin	(intact, no rashes/lesions/erythema)

Physical exam additional notes:

Labs:

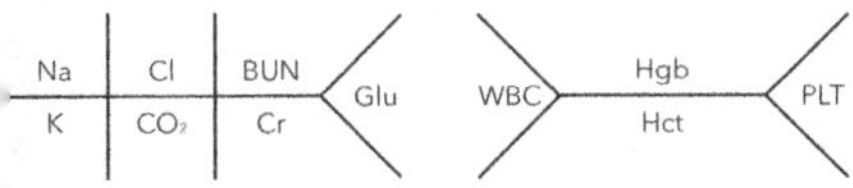

Other Labs:

Studies: (EKG, CXR, other imaging studies)

Impression / Assessment:

Differential Diagnosis:

Plan:

Updates / Notes:

To Do:

Date: Patient Name: Age: Gender:

DOA: Room #: Bed:

Chief Complaint:

History of Present Illness:

Past Medical History: (HTN/DM/CAD/CVA)

Medications:

Past Surgical History:

Family History:

Social History:

Occupation: Lives with: Relationship:

Drug/substance abuse history if any: (alcohol/tobacco/drugs)

Allergies:

Review of Systems: (Describe if not WNL)

General	☐ WNL / ☐ Other	**GI**	☐ WNL / ☐ Other
Skin	☐ WNL / ☐ Other	**GU**	☐ WNL / ☐ Other
ENT	☐ WNL / ☐ Other	**MSK**	☐ WNL / ☐ Other
Eyes	☐ WNL / ☐ Other	**Neuro**	☐ WNL / ☐ Other
CV	☐ WNL / ☐ Other	**Endo**	☐ WNL / ☐ Other
Resp	☐ WNL / ☐ Other	**Psych**	☐ WNL / ☐ Other

ROS additional notes

Physical Exam:

Vitals:	Pulse:	BP:	RR:	Temp:
	SaO_2:	Height:	Weight:	BMI:

General	(NAD, alert, interactive)
HEENT	(NC/AT, MMM, PERRL, EOMI, BL TM intact and reactive to light, BL sclera anicteric)
Neck	(supple, no LAD, no JVD, no thyromegaly)
Cardiovascular	(RRR, S1/S2 normal, no m/r/g)
Respiratory	(CTAB, no r/r/w)
Abdominal	(soft, ND/NT, no masses, normal bowel sounds)
Neurologic	(no focal deficit, CN II-XII intact)
Extremities	(normal tone and ROM)
Skin	(intact, no rashes/lesions/erythema)

Physical exam additional notes:

Labs:

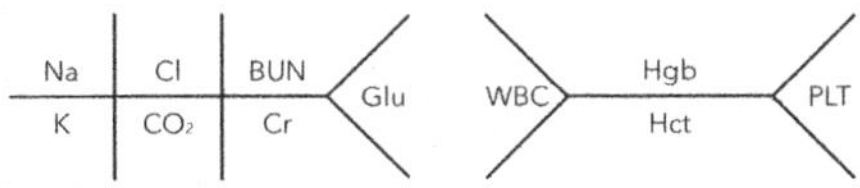

Other Labs:

Studies: (EKG, CXR, other imaging studies)

Impression / Assessment:

Differential Diagnosis:

Plan:

Updates / Notes:

To Do:

Date: Patient Name: Age: Gender:

DOA: Room #: Bed:

Chief Complaint:

History of Present Illness:

Past Medical History: (HTN/DM/CAD/CVA)

Medications:

Past Surgical History:

Family History:

Social History:

Occupation: Lives with: Relationship:

Drug/substance abuse history if any: (alcohol/tobacco/drugs)

Allergies:

Review of Systems: (Describe if not WNL)

General	☐ WNL / ☐ Other	**GI**	☐ WNL / ☐ Other
Skin	☐ WNL / ☐ Other	**GU**	☐ WNL / ☐ Other
ENT	☐ WNL / ☐ Other	**MSK**	☐ WNL / ☐ Other
Eyes	☐ WNL / ☐ Other	**Neuro**	☐ WNL / ☐ Other
CV	☐ WNL / ☐ Other	**Endo**	☐ WNL / ☐ Other
Resp	☐ WNL / ☐ Other	**Psych**	☐ WNL / ☐ Other

ROS additional notes

Physical Exam:

Vitals: Pulse: BP: RR: Temp:

SaO_2: Height: Weight: BMI:

General	(NAD, alert, interactive)
HEENT	(NC/AT, MMM, PERRL, EOMI, BL TM intact and reactive to light, BL sclera anicteric)
Neck	(supple, no LAD, no JVD, no thyromegaly)
Cardiovascular	(RRR, S1/S2 normal, no m/r/g)
Respiratory	(CTAB, no r/r/w)
Abdominal	(soft, ND/NT, no masses, normal bowel sounds)
Neurologic	(no focal deficit, CN II-XII intact)
Extremities	(normal tone and ROM)
Skin	(intact, no rashes/lesions/erythema)

Physical exam additional notes:

Labs:

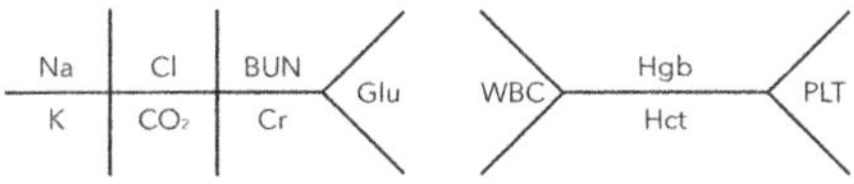

Other Labs:

Studies: (EKG, CXR, other imaging studies)

Impression / Assessment:

Differential Diagnosis:

Plan:

Updates / Notes:

To Do:

Date: Patient Name: Age: Gender:

DOA: Room #: Bed:

Chief Complaint:

History of Present Illness:

Past Medical History: (HTN/DM/CAD/CVA)

Medications:

Past Surgical History:

Family History:

Social History:

Occupation: Lives with: Relationship:

Drug/substance abuse history if any: (alcohol/tobacco/drugs)

Allergies:

Review of Systems: (Describe if not WNL)

General	☐ WNL / ☐ Other	**GI**	☐ WNL / ☐ Other
Skin	☐ WNL / ☐ Other	**GU**	☐ WNL / ☐ Other
ENT	☐ WNL / ☐ Other	**MSK**	☐ WNL / ☐ Other
Eyes	☐ WNL / ☐ Other	**Neuro**	☐ WNL / ☐ Other
CV	☐ WNL / ☐ Other	**Endo**	☐ WNL / ☐ Other
Resp	☐ WNL / ☐ Other	**Psych**	☐ WNL / ☐ Other

ROS additional notes

Physical Exam:

Vitals:	Pulse:	BP:	RR:	Temp:
	SaO_2:	Height:	Weight:	BMI:

General	(NAD, alert, interactive)
HEENT	(NC/AT, MMM, PERRL, EOMI, BL TM intact and reactive to light, BL sclera anicteric)
Neck	(supple, no LAD, no JVD, no thyromegaly)
Cardiovascular	(RRR, S1/S2 normal, no m/r/g)
Respiratory	(CTAB, no r/r/w)
Abdominal	(soft, ND/NT, no masses, normal bowel sounds)
Neurologic	(no focal deficit, CN II-XII intact)
Extremities	(normal tone and ROM)
Skin	(intact, no rashes/lesions/erythema)

Physical exam additional notes:

Labs:

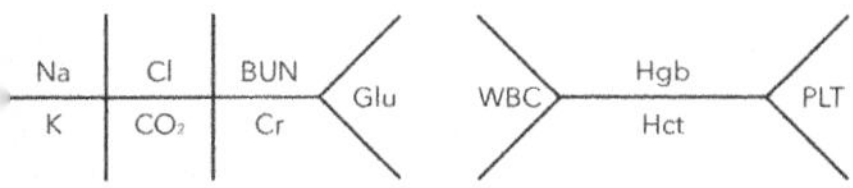

Other Labs:

Studies: (EKG, CXR, other imaging studies)

Impression / Assessment:

Differential Diagnosis:

Plan:

Updates / Notes:

To Do:

Date: Patient Name: Age: Gender:

DOA: Room #: Bed:

Chief Complaint:

History of Present Illness:

Past Medical History: (HTN/DM/CAD/CVA)

Medications:

Past Surgical History:

Family History:

Social History:

Occupation: Lives with: Relationship:

Drug/substance abuse history if any: (alcohol/tobacco/drugs)

Allergies:

Review of Systems: (Describe if not WNL)

General	☐ WNL / ☐ Other	**GI**	☐ WNL / ☐ Other
Skin	☐ WNL / ☐ Other	**GU**	☐ WNL / ☐ Other
ENT	☐ WNL / ☐ Other	**MSK**	☐ WNL / ☐ Other
Eyes	☐ WNL / ☐ Other	**Neuro**	☐ WNL / ☐ Other
CV	☐ WNL / ☐ Other	**Endo**	☐ WNL / ☐ Other
Resp	☐ WNL / ☐ Other	**Psych**	☐ WNL / ☐ Other

ROS additional notes

Physical Exam:

Vitals:	Pulse:	BP:	RR:	Temp:
	SaO_2:	Height:	Weight:	BMI:

General	(NAD, alert, interactive)
HEENT	(NC/AT, MMM, PERRL, EOMI, BL TM intact and reactive to light, BL sclera anicteric)
Neck	(supple, no LAD, no JVD, no thyromegaly)
Cardiovascular	(RRR, S1/S2 normal, no m/r/g)
Respiratory	(CTAB, no r/r/w)
Abdominal	(soft, ND/NT, no masses, normal bowel sounds)
Neurologic	(no focal deficit, CN II-XII intact)
Extremities	(normal tone and ROM)
Skin	(intact, no rashes/lesions/erythema)

Physical exam additional notes:

Labs:

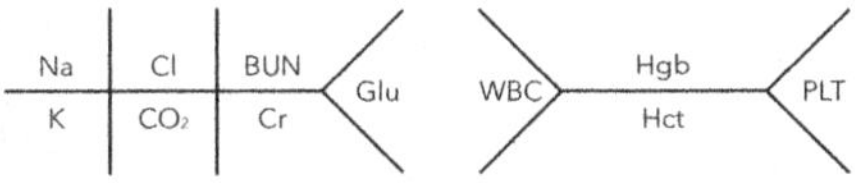

Other Labs:

Studies: (EKG, CXR, other imaging studies)

Impression / Assessment:

Differential Diagnosis:

Plan:

Updates / Notes:

To Do:

Date: Patient Name: Age: Gender:

DOA: Room #: Bed:

Chief Complaint:

History of Present Illness:

Past Medical History: (HTN/DM/CAD/CVA)

Medications:

Past Surgical History:	**Family History:**

Social History:

Occupation: Lives with: Relationship:

Drug/substance abuse history if any: (alcohol/tobacco/drugs)

Allergies:

Review of Systems: (Describe if not WNL)

General	☐ WNL / ☐ Other	**GI**	☐ WNL / ☐ Other
Skin	☐ WNL / ☐ Other	**GU**	☐ WNL / ☐ Other
ENT	☐ WNL / ☐ Other	**MSK**	☐ WNL / ☐ Other
Eyes	☐ WNL / ☐ Other	**Neuro**	☐ WNL / ☐ Other
CV	☐ WNL / ☐ Other	**Endo**	☐ WNL / ☐ Other
Resp	☐ WNL / ☐ Other	**Psych**	☐ WNL / ☐ Other

ROS additional notes

Physical Exam:

Vitals: Pulse: BP: RR: Temp:
SaO$_2$: Height: Weight: BMI:

General	(NAD, alert, interactive)
HEENT	(NC/AT, MMM, PERRL, EOMI, BL TM intact and reactive to light, BL sclera anicteric)
Neck	(supple, no LAD, no JVD, no thyromegaly)
Cardiovascular	(RRR, S1/S2 normal, no m/r/g)
Respiratory	(CTAB, no r/r/w)
Abdominal	(soft, ND/NT, no masses, normal bowel sounds)
Neurologic	(no focal deficit, CN II-XII intact)
Extremities	(normal tone and ROM)
Skin	(intact, no rashes/lesions/erythema)

Physical exam additional notes:

Labs:

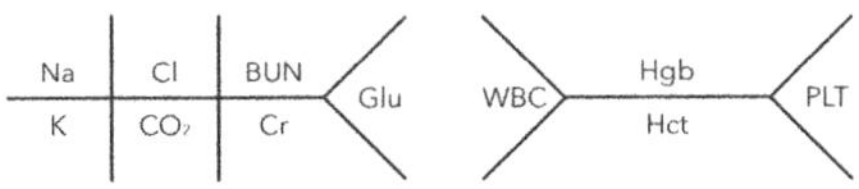

Other Labs:

Studies: (EKG, CXR, other imaging studies)

Impression / Assessment:

Differential Diagnosis:

Plan:

Updates / Notes:

To Do:

Date: Patient Name: Age: Gender:

DOA: Room #: Bed:

Chief Complaint:

History of Present Illness:

Past Medical History: (HTN/DM/CAD/CVA)

Medications:

Past Surgical History:

Family History:

Social History:

Occupation: Lives with: Relationship:

Drug/substance abuse history if any: (alcohol/tobacco/drugs)

Allergies:

Review of Systems: (Describe if not WNL)

General	☐ WNL / ☐ Other	**GI**	☐ WNL / ☐ Other
Skin	☐ WNL / ☐ Other	**GU**	☐ WNL / ☐ Other
ENT	☐ WNL / ☐ Other	**MSK**	☐ WNL / ☐ Other
Eyes	☐ WNL / ☐ Other	**Neuro**	☐ WNL / ☐ Other
CV	☐ WNL / ☐ Other	**Endo**	☐ WNL / ☐ Other
Resp	☐ WNL / ☐ Other	**Psych**	☐ WNL / ☐ Other

ROS additional notes

Physical Exam:

Vitals: Pulse: BP: RR: Temp:
SaO_2: Height: Weight: BMI:

General	(NAD, alert, interactive)
HEENT	(NC/AT, MMM, PERRL, EOMI, BL TM intact and reactive to light, BL sclera anicteric)
Neck	(supple, no LAD, no JVD, no thyromegaly)
Cardiovascular	(RRR, S1/S2 normal, no m/r/g)
Respiratory	(CTAB, no r/r/w)
Abdominal	(soft, ND/NT, no masses, normal bowel sounds)
Neurologic	(no focal deficit, CN II-XII intact)
Extremities	(normal tone and ROM)
Skin	(intact, no rashes/lesions/erythema)

Physical exam additional notes:

Labs:

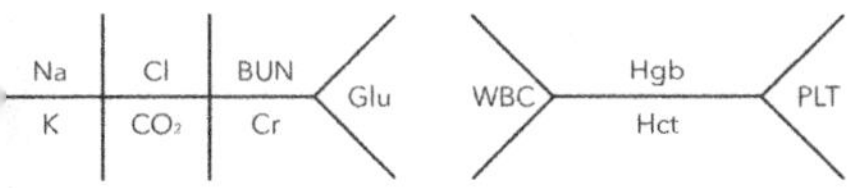

Other Labs:

Studies: (EKG, CXR, other imaging studies)

Impression / Assessment:

Differential Diagnosis:

Plan:

Updates / Notes:

To Do:

Date: Patient Name: Age: Gender:

DOA: Room #: Bed:

Chief Complaint:

History of Present Illness:

Past Medical History: (HTN/DM/CAD/CVA)

Medications:

Past Surgical History:

Family History:

Social History:

Occupation: Lives with: Relationship:

Drug/substance abuse history if any: (alcohol/tobacco/drugs)

Allergies:

Review of Systems: (Describe if not WNL)

General	☐ WNL / ☐ Other	**GI**	☐ WNL / ☐ Other
Skin	☐ WNL / ☐ Other	**GU**	☐ WNL / ☐ Other
ENT	☐ WNL / ☐ Other	**MSK**	☐ WNL / ☐ Other
Eyes	☐ WNL / ☐ Other	**Neuro**	☐ WNL / ☐ Other
CV	☐ WNL / ☐ Other	**Endo**	☐ WNL / ☐ Other
Resp	☐ WNL / ☐ Other	**Psych**	☐ WNL / ☐ Other

ROS additional notes

Physical Exam:

Vitals: Pulse: BP: RR: Temp:

SaO$_2$: Height: Weight: BMI:

General	(NAD, alert, interactive)
HEENT	(NC/AT, MMM, PERRL, EOMI, BL TM intact and reactive to light, BL sclera anicteric)
Neck	(supple, no LAD, no JVD, no thyromegaly)
Cardiovascular	(RRR, S1/S2 normal, no m/r/g)
Respiratory	(CTAB, no r/r/w)
Abdominal	(soft, ND/NT, no masses, normal bowel sounds)
Neurologic	(no focal deficit, CN II-XII intact)
Extremities	(normal tone and ROM)
Skin	(intact, no rashes/lesions/erythema)

Physical exam additional notes:

Labs:

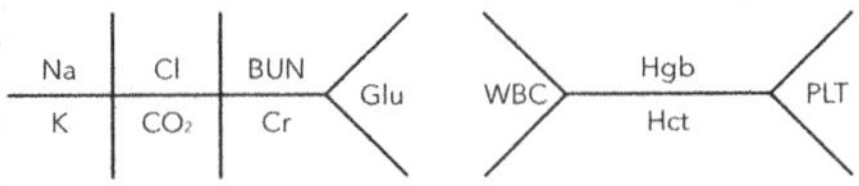

Other Labs:

Studies: (EKG, CXR, other imaging studies)

Impression / Assessment:

Differential Diagnosis:

Plan:

Updates / Notes:

To Do:

Date: Patient Name: Age: Gender:

DOA: Room #: Bed:

Chief Complaint:

History of Present Illness:

Past Medical History: (HTN/DM/CAD/CVA)

Medications:

Past Surgical History:

Family History:

Social History:

Occupation: Lives with: Relationship:

Drug/substance abuse history if any: (alcohol/tobacco/drugs)

Allergies:

Review of Systems: (Describe if not WNL)

General	☐ WNL / ☐ Other	**GI**	☐ WNL / ☐ Other
Skin	☐ WNL / ☐ Other	**GU**	☐ WNL / ☐ Other
ENT	☐ WNL / ☐ Other	**MSK**	☐ WNL / ☐ Other
Eyes	☐ WNL / ☐ Other	**Neuro**	☐ WNL / ☐ Other
CV	☐ WNL / ☐ Other	**Endo**	☐ WNL / ☐ Other
Resp	☐ WNL / ☐ Other	**Psych**	☐ WNL / ☐ Other

ROS additional notes

Physical Exam:

Vitals: Pulse: BP: RR: Temp:
SaO_2: Height: Weight: BMI:

General	(NAD, alert, interactive)
HEENT	(NC/AT, MMM, PERRL, EOMI, BL TM intact and reactive to light, BL sclera anicteric)
Neck	(supple, no LAD, no JVD, no thyromegaly)
Cardiovascular	(RRR, S1/S2 normal, no m/r/g)
Respiratory	(CTAB, no r/r/w)
Abdominal	(soft, ND/NT, no masses, normal bowel sounds)
Neurologic	(no focal deficit, CN II-XII intact)
Extremities	(normal tone and ROM)
Skin	(intact, no rashes/lesions/erythema)

Physical exam additional notes:

Labs:

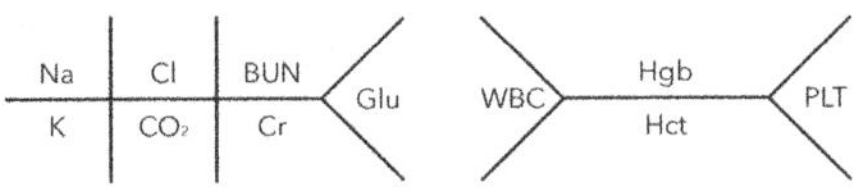

Other Labs:

Studies: (EKG, CXR, other imaging studies)

Impression / Assessment:

Differential Diagnosis:

Plan:

Updates / Notes:

To Do:

Date: Patient Name: Age: Gender:

DOA: Room #: Bed:

Chief Complaint:

History of Present Illness:

Past Medical History: (HTN/DM/CAD/CVA)

Medications:

Past Surgical History:

Family History:

Social History:

Occupation: Lives with: Relationship:

Drug/substance abuse history if any: (alcohol/tobacco/drugs)

Allergies:

Review of Systems: (Describe if not WNL)

General	☐ WNL / ☐ Other	**GI**	☐ WNL / ☐ Other
Skin	☐ WNL / ☐ Other	**GU**	☐ WNL / ☐ Other
ENT	☐ WNL / ☐ Other	**MSK**	☐ WNL / ☐ Other
Eyes	☐ WNL / ☐ Other	**Neuro**	☐ WNL / ☐ Other
CV	☐ WNL / ☐ Other	**Endo**	☐ WNL / ☐ Other
Resp	☐ WNL / ☐ Other	**Psych**	☐ WNL / ☐ Other

ROS additional notes

Physical Exam:

Vitals:	Pulse:	BP:	RR:	Temp:
	SaO_2:	Height:	Weight:	BMI:

General	(NAD, alert, interactive)
HEENT	(NC/AT, MMM, PERRL, EOMI, BL TM intact and reactive to light, BL sclera anicteric)
Neck	(supple, no LAD, no JVD, no thyromegaly)
Cardiovascular	(RRR, S1/S2 normal, no m/r/g)
Respiratory	(CTAB, no r/r/w)
Abdominal	(soft, ND/NT, no masses, normal bowel sounds)
Neurologic	(no focal deficit, CN II-XII intact)
Extremities	(normal tone and ROM)
Skin	(intact, no rashes/lesions/erythema)

Physical exam additional notes:

Labs:

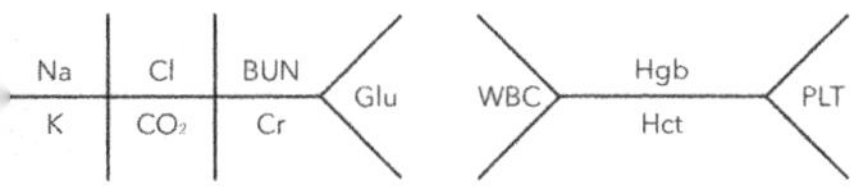

Other Labs:

Studies: (EKG, CXR, other imaging studies)

Impression / Assessment:

Differential Diagnosis:

Plan:

Updates / Notes:

To Do:

Date: Patient Name: Age: Gender:

DOA: Room #: Bed:

Chief Complaint:

History of Present Illness:

Past Medical History: (HTN/DM/CAD/CVA)

Medications:

Past Surgical History:

Family History:

Social History:

Occupation: Lives with: Relationship:

Drug/substance abuse history if any: (alcohol/tobacco/drugs)

Allergies:

Review of Systems: (Describe if not WNL)

General	☐ WNL / ☐ Other	**GI**	☐ WNL / ☐ Other
Skin	☐ WNL / ☐ Other	**GU**	☐ WNL / ☐ Other
ENT	☐ WNL / ☐ Other	**MSK**	☐ WNL / ☐ Other
Eyes	☐ WNL / ☐ Other	**Neuro**	☐ WNL / ☐ Other
CV	☐ WNL / ☐ Other	**Endo**	☐ WNL / ☐ Other
Resp	☐ WNL / ☐ Other	**Psych**	☐ WNL / ☐ Other

ROS additional notes

Physical Exam:

Vitals:	Pulse:	BP:	RR:	Temp:
	SaO_2:	Height:	Weight:	BMI:

General	(NAD, alert, interactive)
HEENT	(NC/AT, MMM, PERRL, EOMI, BL TM intact and reactive to light, BL sclera anicteric)
Neck	(supple, no LAD, no JVD, no thyromegaly)
Cardiovascular	(RRR, S1/S2 normal, no m/r/g)
Respiratory	(CTAB, no r/r/w)
Abdominal	(soft, ND/NT, no masses, normal bowel sounds)
Neurologic	(no focal deficit, CN II-XII intact)
Extremities	(normal tone and ROM)
Skin	(intact, no rashes/lesions/erythema)

Physical exam additional notes:

Labs:

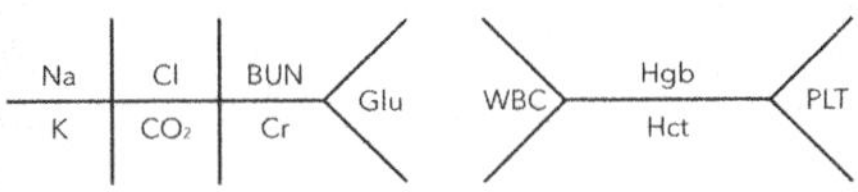

Other Labs:

Studies: (EKG, CXR, other imaging studies)

Impression / Assessment:

Differential Diagnosis:

Plan:

Updates / Notes:

To Do:

Date: Patient Name: Age: Gender:

DOA: Room #: Bed:

Chief Complaint:

History of Present Illness:

Past Medical History: (HTN/DM/CAD/CVA)

Medications:

Past Surgical History:

Family History:

Social History:

Occupation: Lives with: Relationship:

Drug/substance abuse history if any: (alcohol/tobacco/drugs)

Allergies:

Review of Systems: (Describe if not WNL)

General	☐ WNL / ☐ Other	**GI**	☐ WNL / ☐ Other
Skin	☐ WNL / ☐ Other	**GU**	☐ WNL / ☐ Other
ENT	☐ WNL / ☐ Other	**MSK**	☐ WNL / ☐ Other
Eyes	☐ WNL / ☐ Other	**Neuro**	☐ WNL / ☐ Other
CV	☐ WNL / ☐ Other	**Endo**	☐ WNL / ☐ Other
Resp	☐ WNL / ☐ Other	**Psych**	☐ WNL / ☐ Other

ROS additional notes

Physical Exam:

Vitals: Pulse: BP: RR: Temp:
SaO$_2$: Height: Weight: BMI:

General	(NAD, alert, interactive)
HEENT	(NC/AT, MMM, PERRL, EOMI, BL TM intact and reactive to light, BL sclera anicteric)
Neck	(supple, no LAD, no JVD, no thyromegaly)
Cardiovascular	(RRR, S1/S2 normal, no m/r/g)
Respiratory	(CTAB, no r/r/w)
Abdominal	(soft, ND/NT, no masses, normal bowel sounds)
Neurologic	(no focal deficit, CN II-XII intact)
Extremities	(normal tone and ROM)
Skin	(intact, no rashes/lesions/erythema)

Physical exam additional notes:

Labs:

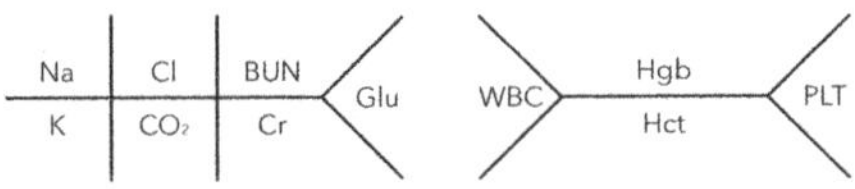

Other Labs:

Studies: (EKG, CXR, other imaging studies)

Impression / Assessment:

Differential Diagnosis:

Plan:

Updates / Notes:

To Do:

Date: Patient Name: Age: Gender:

DOA: Room #: Bed:

Chief Complaint:

History of Present Illness:

Past Medical History: (HTN/DM/CAD/CVA)

Medications:

Past Surgical History:

Family History:

Social History:

Occupation: Lives with: Relationship:

Drug/substance abuse history if any: (alcohol/tobacco/drugs)

Allergies:

Review of Systems: (Describe if not WNL)

General	☐ WNL / ☐ Other	**GI**	☐ WNL / ☐ Other
Skin	☐ WNL / ☐ Other	**GU**	☐ WNL / ☐ Other
ENT	☐ WNL / ☐ Other	**MSK**	☐ WNL / ☐ Other
Eyes	☐ WNL / ☐ Other	**Neuro**	☐ WNL / ☐ Other
CV	☐ WNL / ☐ Other	**Endo**	☐ WNL / ☐ Other
Resp	☐ WNL / ☐ Other	**Psych**	☐ WNL / ☐ Other

ROS additional notes

Physical Exam:

Vitals: Pulse: BP: RR: Temp:

SaO$_2$: Height: Weight: BMI:

General	(NAD, alert, interactive)
HEENT	(NC/AT, MMM, PERRL, EOMI, BL TM intact and reactive to light, BL sclera anicteric)
Neck	(supple, no LAD, no JVD, no thyromegaly)
Cardiovascular	(RRR, S1/S2 normal, no m/r/g)
Respiratory	(CTAB, no r/r/w)
Abdominal	(soft, ND/NT, no masses, normal bowel sounds)
Neurologic	(no focal deficit, CN II-XII intact)
Extremities	(normal tone and ROM)
Skin	(intact, no rashes/lesions/erythema)

Physical exam additional notes:

Labs:

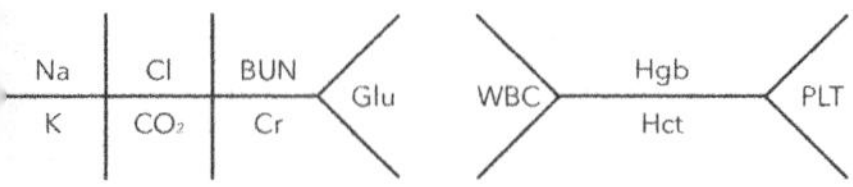

Other Labs:

Studies: (EKG, CXR, other imaging studies)

Impression / Assessment:

Differential Diagnosis:

Plan:

Updates / Notes:

To Do:

Date: Patient Name: Age: Gender:

DOA: Room #: Bed:

Chief Complaint:

History of Present Illness:

Past Medical History: (HTN/DM/CAD/CVA)

Medications:

Past Surgical History:	**Family History:**

Social History:

Occupation: Lives with: Relationship:

Drug/substance abuse history if any: (alcohol/tobacco/drugs)

Allergies:

Review of Systems: (Describe if not WNL)

General	☐ WNL / ☐ Other	**GI**	☐ WNL / ☐ Other
Skin	☐ WNL / ☐ Other	**GU**	☐ WNL / ☐ Other
ENT	☐ WNL / ☐ Other	**MSK**	☐ WNL / ☐ Other
Eyes	☐ WNL / ☐ Other	**Neuro**	☐ WNL / ☐ Other
CV	☐ WNL / ☐ Other	**Endo**	☐ WNL / ☐ Other
Resp	☐ WNL / ☐ Other	**Psych**	☐ WNL / ☐ Other

ROS additional notes

Physical Exam:

Vitals:	Pulse:	BP:	RR:	Temp:
	SaO_2:	Height:	Weight:	BMI:

General	(NAD, alert, interactive)
HEENT	(NC/AT, MMM, PERRL, EOMI, BL TM intact and reactive to light, BL sclera anicteric)
Neck	(supple, no LAD, no JVD, no thyromegaly)
Cardiovascular	(RRR, S1/S2 normal, no m/r/g)
Respiratory	(CTAB, no r/r/w)
Abdominal	(soft, ND/NT, no masses, normal bowel sounds)
Neurologic	(no focal deficit, CN II-XII intact)
Extremities	(normal tone and ROM)
Skin	(intact, no rashes/lesions/erythema)

Physical exam additional notes:

Labs:

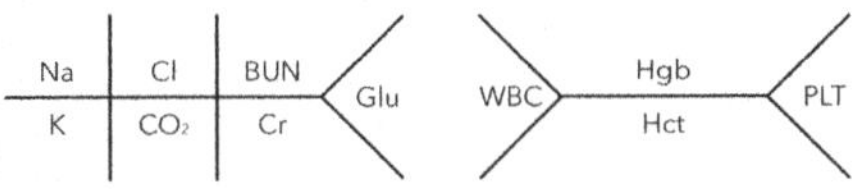

Other Labs:

Studies: (EKG, CXR, other imaging studies)

Impression / Assessment:

Differential Diagnosis:

Plan:

Updates / Notes:

To Do:

Date: Patient Name: Age: Gender:

DOA: Room #: Bed:

Chief Complaint:

History of Present Illness:

Past Medical History: (HTN/DM/CAD/CVA)

Medications:

Past Surgical History:

Family History:

Social History:

Occupation: Lives with: Relationship:

Drug/substance abuse history if any: (alcohol/tobacco/drugs)

Allergies:

Review of Systems: (Describe if not WNL)

General	☐ WNL / ☐ Other	**GI**	☐ WNL / ☐ Other
Skin	☐ WNL / ☐ Other	**GU**	☐ WNL / ☐ Other
ENT	☐ WNL / ☐ Other	**MSK**	☐ WNL / ☐ Other
Eyes	☐ WNL / ☐ Other	**Neuro**	☐ WNL / ☐ Other
CV	☐ WNL / ☐ Other	**Endo**	☐ WNL / ☐ Other
Resp	☐ WNL / ☐ Other	**Psych**	☐ WNL / ☐ Other

ROS additional notes

Physical Exam:

Vitals:	Pulse:	BP:	RR:	Temp:
	SaO_2:	Height:	Weight:	BMI:

General	(NAD, alert, interactive)
HEENT	(NC/AT, MMM, PERRL, EOMI, BL TM intact and reactive to light, BL sclera anicteric)
Neck	(supple, no LAD, no JVD, no thyromegaly)
Cardiovascular	(RRR, S1/S2 normal, no m/r/g)
Respiratory	(CTAB, no r/r/w)
Abdominal	(soft, ND/NT, no masses, normal bowel sounds)
Neurologic	(no focal deficit, CN II-XII intact)
Extremities	(normal tone and ROM)
Skin	(intact, no rashes/lesions/erythema)

Physical exam additional notes:

Labs:

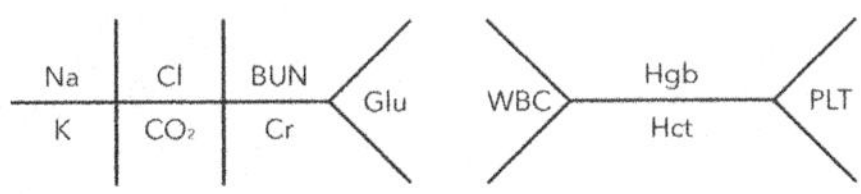

Other Labs:

Studies: (EKG, CXR, other imaging studies)

Impression / Assessment:

Differential Diagnosis:

Plan:

Updates / Notes:

To Do:

Date: Patient Name: Age: Gender:

DOA: Room #: Bed:

Chief Complaint:

History of Present Illness:

Past Medical History: (HTN/DM/CAD/CVA)

Medications:

Past Surgical History:

Family History:

Social History:

Occupation: Lives with: Relationship:

Drug/substance abuse history if any: (alcohol/tobacco/drugs)

Allergies:

Review of Systems: (Describe if not WNL)

General	☐ WNL / ☐ Other	**GI**	☐ WNL / ☐ Other
Skin	☐ WNL / ☐ Other	**GU**	☐ WNL / ☐ Other
ENT	☐ WNL / ☐ Other	**MSK**	☐ WNL / ☐ Other
Eyes	☐ WNL / ☐ Other	**Neuro**	☐ WNL / ☐ Other
CV	☐ WNL / ☐ Other	**Endo**	☐ WNL / ☐ Other
Resp	☐ WNL / ☐ Other	**Psych**	☐ WNL / ☐ Other

ROS additional notes

Physical Exam:

Vitals: Pulse: BP: RR: Temp:
SaO$_2$: Height: Weight: BMI:

General	(NAD, alert, interactive)
HEENT	(NC/AT, MMM, PERRL, EOMI, BL TM intact and reactive to light, BL sclera anicteric)
Neck	(supple, no LAD, no JVD, no thyromegaly)
Cardiovascular	(RRR, S1/S2 normal, no m/r/g)
Respiratory	(CTAB, no r/r/w)
Abdominal	(soft, ND/NT, no masses, normal bowel sounds)
Neurologic	(no focal deficit, CN II-XII intact)
Extremities	(normal tone and ROM)
Skin	(intact, no rashes/lesions/erythema)

Physical exam additional notes:

Labs:

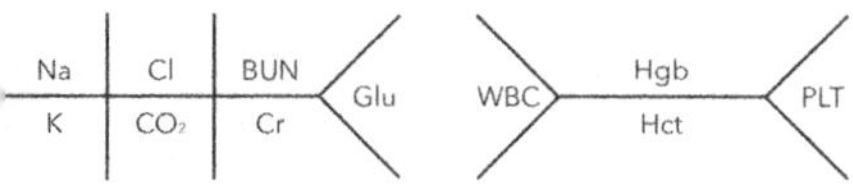

Other Labs:

Studies: (EKG, CXR, other imaging studies)

Impression / Assessment:

Differential Diagnosis:

Plan:

Updates / Notes:

To Do:

Date: Patient Name: Age: Gender:

DOA: Room #: Bed:

Chief Complaint:

History of Present Illness:

Past Medical History: (HTN/DM/CAD/CVA)

Medications:

Past Surgical History:

Family History:

Social History:

Occupation: Lives with: Relationship:

Drug/substance abuse history if any: (alcohol/tobacco/drugs)

Allergies:

Review of Systems: (Describe if not WNL)

General	☐ WNL / ☐ Other	**GI**	☐ WNL / ☐ Other
Skin	☐ WNL / ☐ Other	**GU**	☐ WNL / ☐ Other
ENT	☐ WNL / ☐ Other	**MSK**	☐ WNL / ☐ Other
Eyes	☐ WNL / ☐ Other	**Neuro**	☐ WNL / ☐ Other
CV	☐ WNL / ☐ Other	**Endo**	☐ WNL / ☐ Other
Resp	☐ WNL / ☐ Other	**Psych**	☐ WNL / ☐ Other

ROS additional notes

Physical Exam:

Vitals: Pulse: BP: RR: Temp:
SaO$_2$: Height: Weight: BMI:

General	(NAD, alert, interactive)
HEENT	(NC/AT, MMM, PERRL, EOMI, BL TM intact and reactive to light, BL sclera anicteric)
Neck	(supple, no LAD, no JVD, no thyromegaly)
Cardiovascular	(RRR, S1/S2 normal, no m/r/g)
Respiratory	(CTAB, no r/r/w)
Abdominal	(soft, ND/NT, no masses, normal bowel sounds)
Neurologic	(no focal deficit, CN II-XII intact)
Extremities	(normal tone and ROM)
Skin	(intact, no rashes/lesions/erythema)

Physical exam additional notes:

Labs:

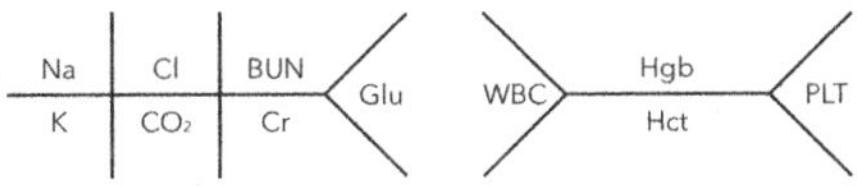

Other Labs:

Studies: (EKG, CXR, other imaging studies)

Impression / Assessment:

Differential Diagnosis:

Plan:

Updates / Notes:

To Do:

Date: Patient Name: Age: Gender:

DOA: Room #: Bed:

Chief Complaint:

History of Present Illness:

Past Medical History: (HTN/DM/CAD/CVA)

Medications:

Past Surgical History:

Family History:

Social History:

Occupation: Lives with: Relationship:

Drug/substance abuse history if any: (alcohol/tobacco/drugs)

Allergies:

Review of Systems: (Describe if not WNL)

General	☐ WNL / ☐ Other	**GI**	☐ WNL / ☐ Other
Skin	☐ WNL / ☐ Other	**GU**	☐ WNL / ☐ Other
ENT	☐ WNL / ☐ Other	**MSK**	☐ WNL / ☐ Other
Eyes	☐ WNL / ☐ Other	**Neuro**	☐ WNL / ☐ Other
CV	☐ WNL / ☐ Other	**Endo**	☐ WNL / ☐ Other
Resp	☐ WNL / ☐ Other	**Psych**	☐ WNL / ☐ Other

ROS additional notes

Physical Exam:

Vitals: Pulse: BP: RR: Temp:
SaO_2: Height: Weight: BMI:

General	(NAD, alert, interactive)
HEENT	(NC/AT, MMM, PERRL, EOMI, BL TM intact and reactive to light, BL sclera anicteric)
Neck	(supple, no LAD, no JVD, no thyromegaly)
Cardiovascular	(RRR, S1/S2 normal, no m/r/g)
Respiratory	(CTAB, no r/r/w)
Abdominal	(soft, ND/NT, no masses, normal bowel sounds)
Neurologic	(no focal deficit, CN II-XII intact)
Extremities	(normal tone and ROM)
Skin	(intact, no rashes/lesions/erythema)

Physical exam additional notes:

Labs:

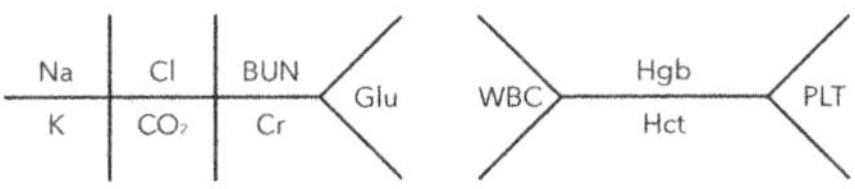

Other Labs:

Studies: (EKG, CXR, other imaging studies)

Impression / Assessment:

Differential Diagnosis:

Plan:

Updates / Notes:

To Do:

Date: Patient Name: Age: Gender:

DOA: Room #: Bed:

Chief Complaint:

History of Present Illness:

Past Medical History: (HTN/DM/CAD/CVA)

Medications:

Past Surgical History:

Family History:

Social History:

Occupation: Lives with: Relationship:

Drug/substance abuse history if any: (alcohol/tobacco/drugs)

Allergies:

Review of Systems: (Describe if not WNL)

General	☐ WNL / ☐ Other	**GI**	☐ WNL / ☐ Other
Skin	☐ WNL / ☐ Other	**GU**	☐ WNL / ☐ Other
ENT	☐ WNL / ☐ Other	**MSK**	☐ WNL / ☐ Other
Eyes	☐ WNL / ☐ Other	**Neuro**	☐ WNL / ☐ Other
CV	☐ WNL / ☐ Other	**Endo**	☐ WNL / ☐ Other
Resp	☐ WNL / ☐ Other	**Psych**	☐ WNL / ☐ Other

ROS additional notes

hysical Exam:

itals: Pulse: BP: RR: Temp:
SaO2: Height: Weight: BMI:

General	(NAD, alert, interactive)
HEENT	(NC/AT, MMM, PERRL, EOMI, BL TM intact and reactive to light, BL sclera anicteric)
Neck	(supple, no LAD, no JVD, no thyromegaly)
Cardiovascular	(RRR, S1/S2 normal, no m/r/g)
Respiratory	(CTAB, no r/r/w)
Abdominal	(soft, ND/NT, no masses, normal bowel sounds)
Neurologic	(no focal deficit, CN II-XII intact)
Extremities	(normal tone and ROM)
Skin	(intact, no rashes/lesions/erythema)

hysical exam additional notes:

abs:

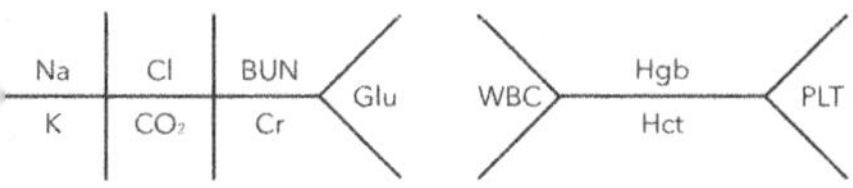

ther Labs:

Studies: (EKG, CXR, other imaging studies)

mpression / Assessment:

ifferential Diagnosis:

lan:

pdates / Notes:

To Do:

Date: Patient Name: Age: Gender:

DOA: Room #: Bed:

Chief Complaint:

History of Present Illness:

Past Medical History: (HTN/DM/CAD/CVA)

Medications:

Past Surgical History:

Family History:

Social History:

Occupation: Lives with: Relationship:

Drug/substance abuse history if any: (alcohol/tobacco/drugs)

Allergies:

Review of Systems: (Describe if not WNL)

General	☐ WNL / ☐ Other	**GI**	☐ WNL / ☐ Other
Skin	☐ WNL / ☐ Other	**GU**	☐ WNL / ☐ Other
ENT	☐ WNL / ☐ Other	**MSK**	☐ WNL / ☐ Other
Eyes	☐ WNL / ☐ Other	**Neuro**	☐ WNL / ☐ Other
CV	☐ WNL / ☐ Other	**Endo**	☐ WNL / ☐ Other
Resp	☐ WNL / ☐ Other	**Psych**	☐ WNL / ☐ Other

ROS additional notes

Physical Exam:

Vitals:	Pulse:	BP:	RR:	Temp:
	SaO_2:	Height:	Weight:	BMI:

General	(NAD, alert, interactive)
HEENT	(NC/AT, MMM, PERRL, EOMI, BL TM intact and reactive to light, BL sclera anicteric)
Neck	(supple, no LAD, no JVD, no thyromegaly)
Cardiovascular	(RRR, S1/S2 normal, no m/r/g)
Respiratory	(CTAB, no r/r/w)
Abdominal	(soft, ND/NT, no masses, normal bowel sounds)
Neurologic	(no focal deficit, CN II-XII intact)
Extremities	(normal tone and ROM)
Skin	(intact, no rashes/lesions/erythema)

Physical exam additional notes:

Labs:

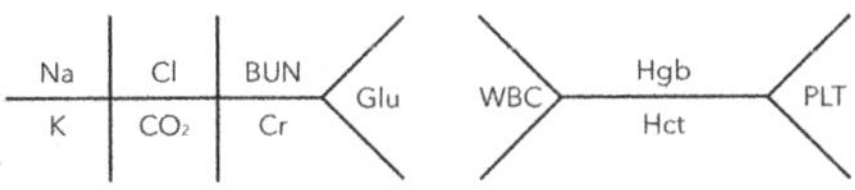

Other Labs:

Studies: (EKG, CXR, other imaging studies)

Impression / Assessment:

Differential Diagnosis:

Plan:

Updates / Notes:

To Do:

Date: Patient Name: Age: Gender:

DOA: Room #: Bed:

Chief Complaint:

History of Present Illness:

Past Medical History: (HTN/DM/CAD/CVA)

Medications:

Past Surgical History:

Family History:

Social History:

Occupation: Lives with: Relationship:

Drug/substance abuse history if any: (alcohol/tobacco/drugs)

Allergies:

Review of Systems: (Describe if not WNL)

General	☐ WNL / ☐ Other	**GI**	☐ WNL / ☐ Other
Skin	☐ WNL / ☐ Other	**GU**	☐ WNL / ☐ Other
ENT	☐ WNL / ☐ Other	**MSK**	☐ WNL / ☐ Other
Eyes	☐ WNL / ☐ Other	**Neuro**	☐ WNL / ☐ Other
CV	☐ WNL / ☐ Other	**Endo**	☐ WNL / ☐ Other
Resp	☐ WNL / ☐ Other	**Psych**	☐ WNL / ☐ Other

ROS additional notes

Physical Exam:

Vitals: Pulse: BP: RR: Temp:
SaO_2: Height: Weight: BMI:

General	(NAD, alert, interactive)
HEENT	(NC/AT, MMM, PERRL, EOMI, BL TM intact and reactive to light, BL sclera anicteric)
Neck	(supple, no LAD, no JVD, no thyromegaly)
Cardiovascular	(RRR, S1/S2 normal, no m/r/g)
Respiratory	(CTAB, no r/r/w)
Abdominal	(soft, ND/NT, no masses, normal bowel sounds)
Neurologic	(no focal deficit, CN II-XII intact)
Extremities	(normal tone and ROM)
Skin	(intact, no rashes/lesions/erythema)

Physical exam additional notes:

Labs:

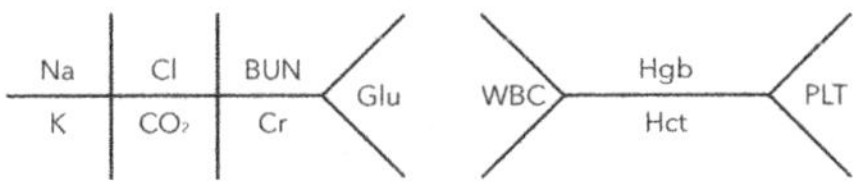

Other Labs:

Studies: (EKG, CXR, other imaging studies)

Impression / Assessment:

Differential Diagnosis:

Plan:

Updates / Notes:

To Do:

Date: Patient Name: Age: Gender:

DOA: Room #: Bed:

Chief Complaint:

History of Present Illness:

Past Medical History: (HTN/DM/CAD/CVA)

Medications:

Past Surgical History:

Family History:

Social History:

Occupation: Lives with: Relationship:

Drug/substance abuse history if any: (alcohol/tobacco/drugs)

Allergies:

Review of Systems: (Describe if not WNL)

General	☐ WNL / ☐ Other	**GI**	☐ WNL / ☐ Other
Skin	☐ WNL / ☐ Other	**GU**	☐ WNL / ☐ Other
ENT	☐ WNL / ☐ Other	**MSK**	☐ WNL / ☐ Other
Eyes	☐ WNL / ☐ Other	**Neuro**	☐ WNL / ☐ Other
CV	☐ WNL / ☐ Other	**Endo**	☐ WNL / ☐ Other
Resp	☐ WNL / ☐ Other	**Psych**	☐ WNL / ☐ Other

ROS additional notes

Physical Exam:

Vitals: Pulse: BP: RR: Temp:
SaO2: Height: Weight: BMI:

General	(NAD, alert, interactive)
HEENT	(NC/AT, MMM, PERRL, EOMI, BL TM intact and reactive to light, BL sclera anicteric)
Neck	(supple, no LAD, no JVD, no thyromegaly)
Cardiovascular	(RRR, S1/S2 normal, no m/r/g)
Respiratory	(CTAB, no r/r/w)
Abdominal	(soft, ND/NT, no masses, normal bowel sounds)
Neurologic	(no focal deficit, CN II-XII intact)
Extremities	(normal tone and ROM)
Skin	(intact, no rashes/lesions/erythema)

Physical exam additional notes:

Labs:

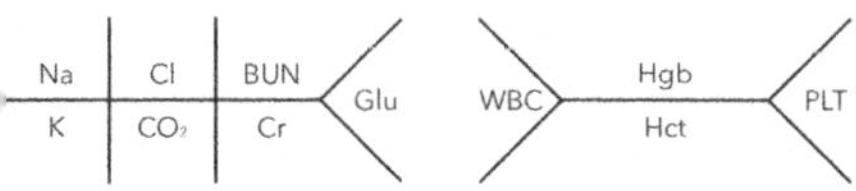

Other Labs:

Studies: (EKG, CXR, other imaging studies)

Impression / Assessment:

Differential Diagnosis:

Plan:

Updates / Notes:

To Do:

Date: Patient Name: Age: Gender:

DOA: Room #: Bed:

Chief Complaint:

History of Present Illness:

Past Medical History: (HTN/DM/CAD/CVA)

Medications:

Past Surgical History:

Family History:

Social History:

Occupation: Lives with: Relationship:

Drug/substance abuse history if any: (alcohol/tobacco/drugs)

Allergies:

Review of Systems: (Describe if not WNL)

General	☐ WNL / ☐ Other	**GI**	☐ WNL / ☐ Other
Skin	☐ WNL / ☐ Other	**GU**	☐ WNL / ☐ Other
ENT	☐ WNL / ☐ Other	**MSK**	☐ WNL / ☐ Other
Eyes	☐ WNL / ☐ Other	**Neuro**	☐ WNL / ☐ Other
CV	☐ WNL / ☐ Other	**Endo**	☐ WNL / ☐ Other
Resp	☐ WNL / ☐ Other	**Psych**	☐ WNL / ☐ Other

ROS additional notes

Physical Exam:

Vitals:	Pulse:	BP:	RR:	Temp:
	SaO_2:	Height:	Weight:	BMI:

General	(NAD, alert, interactive)
HEENT	(NC/AT, MMM, PERRL, EOMI, BL TM intact and reactive to light, BL sclera anicteric)
Neck	(supple, no LAD, no JVD, no thyromegaly)
Cardiovascular	(RRR, S1/S2 normal, no m/r/g)
Respiratory	(CTAB, no r/r/w)
Abdominal	(soft, ND/NT, no masses, normal bowel sounds)
Neurologic	(no focal deficit, CN II-XII intact)
Extremities	(normal tone and ROM)
Skin	(intact, no rashes/lesions/erythema)

Physical exam additional notes:

Labs:

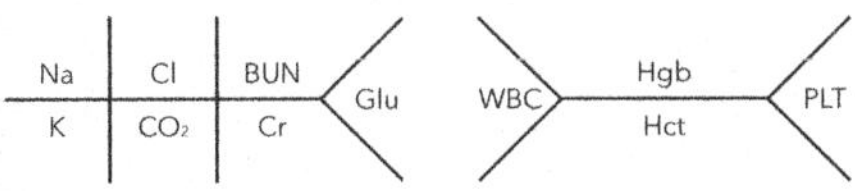

Other Labs:

Studies: (EKG, CXR, other imaging studies)

Impression / Assessment:

Differential Diagnosis:

Plan:

Updates / Notes:

To Do:

Date: Patient Name: Age: Gender:

DOA: Room #: Bed:

Chief Complaint:

History of Present Illness:

Past Medical History: (HTN/DM/CAD/CVA)

Medications:

Past Surgical History:

Family History:

Social History:

Occupation: Lives with: Relationship:

Drug/substance abuse history if any: (alcohol/tobacco/drugs)

Allergies:

Review of Systems: (Describe if not WNL)

General	☐ WNL / ☐ Other	**GI**	☐ WNL / ☐ Other
Skin	☐ WNL / ☐ Other	**GU**	☐ WNL / ☐ Other
ENT	☐ WNL / ☐ Other	**MSK**	☐ WNL / ☐ Other
Eyes	☐ WNL / ☐ Other	**Neuro**	☐ WNL / ☐ Other
CV	☐ WNL / ☐ Other	**Endo**	☐ WNL / ☐ Other
Resp	☐ WNL / ☐ Other	**Psych**	☐ WNL / ☐ Other

ROS additional notes

Physical Exam:

Vitals: Pulse: BP: RR: Temp:
SaO_2: Height: Weight: BMI:

General	(NAD, alert, interactive)
HEENT	(NC/AT, MMM, PERRL, EOMI, BL TM intact and reactive to light, BL sclera anicteric)
Neck	(supple, no LAD, no JVD, no thyromegaly)
Cardiovascular	(RRR, S1/S2 normal, no m/r/g)
Respiratory	(CTAB, no r/r/w)
Abdominal	(soft, ND/NT, no masses, normal bowel sounds)
Neurologic	(no focal deficit, CN II-XII intact)
Extremities	(normal tone and ROM)
Skin	(intact, no rashes/lesions/erythema)

Physical exam additional notes:

Labs:

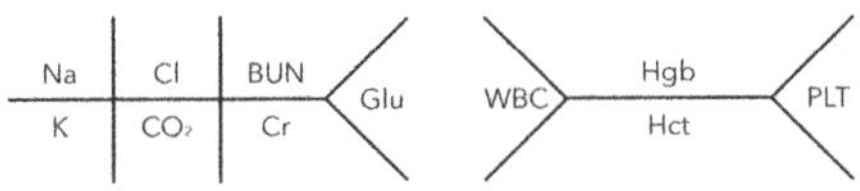

Other Labs:

Studies: (EKG, CXR, other imaging studies)

Impression / Assessment:

Differential Diagnosis:

Plan:

Updates / Notes:

To Do:

Date: Patient Name: Age: Gender:

DOA: Room #: Bed:

Chief Complaint:

History of Present Illness:

Past Medical History: (HTN/DM/CAD/CVA)

Medications:

Past Surgical History:

Family History:

Social History:

Occupation: Lives with: Relationship:

Drug/substance abuse history if any: (alcohol/tobacco/drugs)

Allergies:

Review of Systems: (Describe if not WNL)

General	☐ WNL / ☐ Other	**GI**	☐ WNL / ☐ Other
Skin	☐ WNL / ☐ Other	**GU**	☐ WNL / ☐ Other
ENT	☐ WNL / ☐ Other	**MSK**	☐ WNL / ☐ Other
Eyes	☐ WNL / ☐ Other	**Neuro**	☐ WNL / ☐ Other
CV	☐ WNL / ☐ Other	**Endo**	☐ WNL / ☐ Other
Resp	☐ WNL / ☐ Other	**Psych**	☐ WNL / ☐ Other

ROS additional notes

Physical Exam:

Vitals: Pulse: BP: RR: Temp:

SaO$_2$: Height: Weight: BMI:

General	(NAD, alert, interactive)
HEENT	(NC/AT, MMM, PERRL, EOMI, BL TM intact and reactive to light, BL sclera anicteric)
Neck	(supple, no LAD, no JVD, no thyromegaly)
Cardiovascular	(RRR, S1/S2 normal, no m/r/g)
Respiratory	(CTAB, no r/r/w)
Abdominal	(soft, ND/NT, no masses, normal bowel sounds)
Neurologic	(no focal deficit, CN II-XII intact)
Extremities	(normal tone and ROM)
Skin	(intact, no rashes/lesions/erythema)

Physical exam additional notes:

Labs:

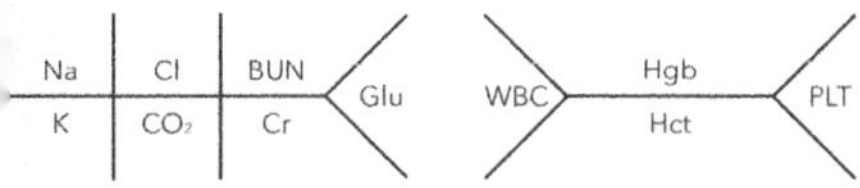

Other Labs:

Studies: (EKG, CXR, other imaging studies)

Impression / Assessment:

Differential Diagnosis:

Plan:

Updates / Notes:

To Do:

Date: Patient Name: Age: Gender:

DOA: Room #: Bed:

Chief Complaint:

History of Present Illness:

Past Medical History: (HTN/DM/CAD/CVA)

Medications:

Past Surgical History:

Family History:

Social History:

Occupation: Lives with: Relationship:

Drug/substance abuse history if any: (alcohol/tobacco/drugs)

Allergies:

Review of Systems: (Describe if not WNL)

General	☐ WNL / ☐ Other	**GI**	☐ WNL / ☐ Other
Skin	☐ WNL / ☐ Other	**GU**	☐ WNL / ☐ Other
ENT	☐ WNL / ☐ Other	**MSK**	☐ WNL / ☐ Other
Eyes	☐ WNL / ☐ Other	**Neuro**	☐ WNL / ☐ Other
CV	☐ WNL / ☐ Other	**Endo**	☐ WNL / ☐ Other
Resp	☐ WNL / ☐ Other	**Psych**	☐ WNL / ☐ Other

ROS additional notes

Physical Exam:

Vitals: Pulse: BP: RR: Temp:
SaO$_2$: Height: Weight: BMI:

General	(NAD, alert, interactive)
HEENT	(NC/AT, MMM, PERRL, EOMI, BL TM intact and reactive to light, BL sclera anicteric)
Neck	(supple, no LAD, no JVD, no thyromegaly)
Cardiovascular	(RRR, S1/S2 normal, no m/r/g)
Respiratory	(CTAB, no r/r/w)
Abdominal	(soft, ND/NT, no masses, normal bowel sounds)
Neurologic	(no focal deficit, CN II-XII intact)
Extremities	(normal tone and ROM)
Skin	(intact, no rashes/lesions/erythema)

Physical exam additional notes:

Labs:

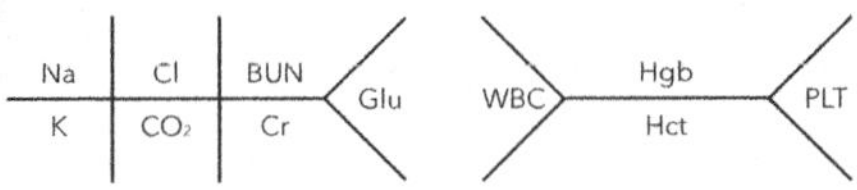

Other Labs:

Studies: (EKG, CXR, other imaging studies)

Impression / Assessment:

Differential Diagnosis:

Plan:

Updates / Notes:

To Do:

Date: Patient Name: Age: Gender:

DOA: Room #: Bed:

Chief Complaint:

History of Present Illness:

Past Medical History: (HTN/DM/CAD/CVA)

Medications:

Past Surgical History:

Family History:

Social History:

Occupation: Lives with: Relationship:

Drug/substance abuse history if any: (alcohol/tobacco/drugs)

Allergies:

Review of Systems: (Describe if not WNL)

General	☐ WNL / ☐ Other	**GI**	☐ WNL / ☐ Other
Skin	☐ WNL / ☐ Other	**GU**	☐ WNL / ☐ Other
ENT	☐ WNL / ☐ Other	**MSK**	☐ WNL / ☐ Other
Eyes	☐ WNL / ☐ Other	**Neuro**	☐ WNL / ☐ Other
CV	☐ WNL / ☐ Other	**Endo**	☐ WNL / ☐ Other
Resp	☐ WNL / ☐ Other	**Psych**	☐ WNL / ☐ Other

ROS additional notes

Physical Exam:

Vitals:	Pulse:	BP:	RR:	Temp:
	SaO_2:	Height:	Weight:	BMI:

General	(NAD, alert, interactive)
HEENT	(NC/AT, MMM, PERRL, EOMI, BL TM intact and reactive to light, BL sclera anicteric)
Neck	(supple, no LAD, no JVD, no thyromegaly)
Cardiovascular	(RRR, S1/S2 normal, no m/r/g)
Respiratory	(CTAB, no r/r/w)
Abdominal	(soft, ND/NT, no masses, normal bowel sounds)
Neurologic	(no focal deficit, CN II-XII intact)
Extremities	(normal tone and ROM)
Skin	(intact, no rashes/lesions/erythema)

Physical exam additional notes:

Labs:

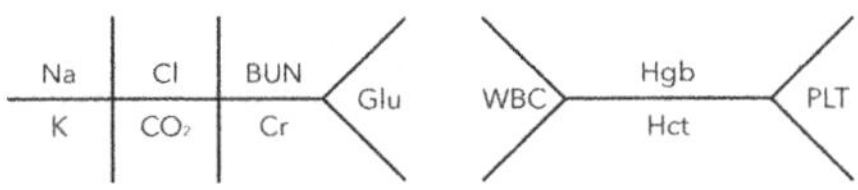

Other Labs:

Studies: (EKG, CXR, other imaging studies)

Impression / Assessment:

Differential Diagnosis:

Plan:

Updates / Notes:

To Do:

Date: Patient Name: Age: Gender:

DOA: Room #: Bed:

Chief Complaint:

History of Present Illness:

Past Medical History: (HTN/DM/CAD/CVA)

Medications:

Past Surgical History:

Family History:

Social History:

Occupation: Lives with: Relationship:

Drug/substance abuse history if any: (alcohol/tobacco/drugs)

Allergies:

Review of Systems: (Describe if not WNL)

General	☐ WNL / ☐ Other	**GI**	☐ WNL / ☐ Other
Skin	☐ WNL / ☐ Other	**GU**	☐ WNL / ☐ Other
ENT	☐ WNL / ☐ Other	**MSK**	☐ WNL / ☐ Other
Eyes	☐ WNL / ☐ Other	**Neuro**	☐ WNL / ☐ Other
CV	☐ WNL / ☐ Other	**Endo**	☐ WNL / ☐ Other
Resp	☐ WNL / ☐ Other	**Psych**	☐ WNL / ☐ Other

ROS additional notes

Physical Exam:

Vitals: Pulse: BP: RR: Temp:

SaO$_2$: Height: Weight: BMI:

General	(NAD, alert, interactive)
HEENT	(NC/AT, MMM, PERRL, EOMI, BL TM intact and reactive to light, BL sclera anicteric)
Neck	(supple, no LAD, no JVD, no thyromegaly)
Cardiovascular	(RRR, S1/S2 normal, no m/r/g)
Respiratory	(CTAB, no r/r/w)
Abdominal	(soft, ND/NT, no masses, normal bowel sounds)
Neurologic	(no focal deficit, CN II-XII intact)
Extremities	(normal tone and ROM)
Skin	(intact, no rashes/lesions/erythema)

Physical exam additional notes:

Labs:

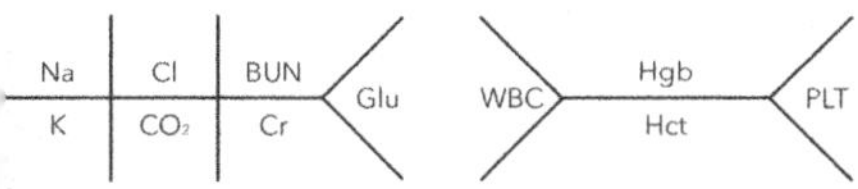

Other Labs:

Studies: (EKG, CXR, other imaging studies)

Impression / Assessment:

Differential Diagnosis:

Plan:

Updates / Notes:

To Do:

Date: Patient Name: Age: Gender:

DOA: Room #: Bed:

Chief Complaint:

History of Present Illness:

Past Medical History: (HTN/DM/CAD/CVA)

Medications:

Past Surgical History:

Family History:

Social History:

Occupation: Lives with: Relationship:

Drug/substance abuse history if any: (alcohol/tobacco/drugs)

Allergies:

Review of Systems: (Describe if not WNL)

General	☐ WNL / ☐ Other	**GI**	☐ WNL / ☐ Other
Skin	☐ WNL / ☐ Other	**GU**	☐ WNL / ☐ Other
ENT	☐ WNL / ☐ Other	**MSK**	☐ WNL / ☐ Other
Eyes	☐ WNL / ☐ Other	**Neuro**	☐ WNL / ☐ Other
CV	☐ WNL / ☐ Other	**Endo**	☐ WNL / ☐ Other
Resp	☐ WNL / ☐ Other	**Psych**	☐ WNL / ☐ Other

ROS additional notes

Physical Exam:

Vitals: Pulse: BP: RR: Temp:

SaO$_2$: Height: Weight: BMI:

General	(NAD, alert, interactive)
HEENT	(NC/AT, MMM, PERRL, EOMI, BL TM intact and reactive to light, BL sclera anicteric)
Neck	(supple, no LAD, no JVD, no thyromegaly)
Cardiovascular	(RRR, S1/S2 normal, no m/r/g)
Respiratory	(CTAB, no r/r/w)
Abdominal	(soft, ND/NT, no masses, normal bowel sounds)
Neurologic	(no focal deficit, CN II-XII intact)
Extremities	(normal tone and ROM)
Skin	(intact, no rashes/lesions/erythema)

Physical exam additional notes:

Labs:

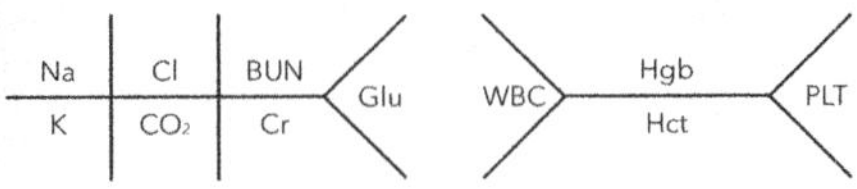

Other Labs:

Studies: (EKG, CXR, other imaging studies)

Impression / Assessment:

Differential Diagnosis:

Plan:

Updates / Notes:

To Do:

Date: Patient Name: Age: Gender:

DOA: Room #: Bed:

Chief Complaint:

History of Present Illness:

Past Medical History: (HTN/DM/CAD/CVA)

Medications:

Past Surgical History:

Family History:

Social History:

Occupation: Lives with: Relationship:

Drug/substance abuse history if any: (alcohol/tobacco/drugs)

Allergies:

Review of Systems: (Describe if not WNL)

General	☐ WNL / ☐ Other	**GI**	☐ WNL / ☐ Other
Skin	☐ WNL / ☐ Other	**GU**	☐ WNL / ☐ Other
ENT	☐ WNL / ☐ Other	**MSK**	☐ WNL / ☐ Other
Eyes	☐ WNL / ☐ Other	**Neuro**	☐ WNL / ☐ Other
CV	☐ WNL / ☐ Other	**Endo**	☐ WNL / ☐ Other
Resp	☐ WNL / ☐ Other	**Psych**	☐ WNL / ☐ Other

ROS additional notes

Physical Exam:

Vitals: Pulse: BP: RR: Temp:
SaO_2: Height: Weight: BMI:

General	(NAD, alert, interactive)
HEENT	(NC/AT, MMM, PERRL, EOMI, BL TM intact and reactive to light, BL sclera anicteric)
Neck	(supple, no LAD, no JVD, no thyromegaly)
Cardiovascular	(RRR, S1/S2 normal, no m/r/g)
Respiratory	(CTAB, no r/r/w)
Abdominal	(soft, ND/NT, no masses, normal bowel sounds)
Neurologic	(no focal deficit, CN II-XII intact)
Extremities	(normal tone and ROM)
Skin	(intact, no rashes/lesions/erythema)

Physical exam additional notes:

Labs:

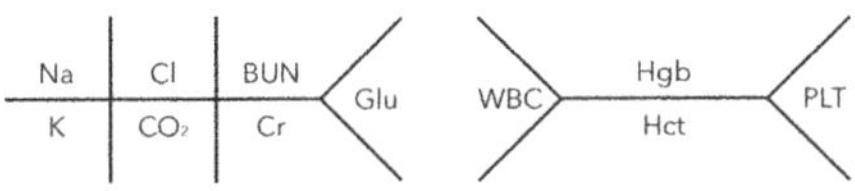

Other Labs:

Studies: (EKG, CXR, other imaging studies)

Impression / Assessment:

Differential Diagnosis:

Plan:

Updates / Notes:

To Do:

Date: Patient Name: Age: Gender:

DOA: Room #: Bed:

Chief Complaint:

History of Present Illness:

Past Medical History: (HTN/DM/CAD/CVA)

Medications:

Past Surgical History:

Family History:

Social History:

Occupation: Lives with: Relationship:

Drug/substance abuse history if any: (alcohol/tobacco/drugs)

Allergies:

Review of Systems: (Describe if not WNL)

General	☐ WNL / ☐ Other	**GI**	☐ WNL / ☐ Other
Skin	☐ WNL / ☐ Other	**GU**	☐ WNL / ☐ Other
ENT	☐ WNL / ☐ Other	**MSK**	☐ WNL / ☐ Other
Eyes	☐ WNL / ☐ Other	**Neuro**	☐ WNL / ☐ Other
CV	☐ WNL / ☐ Other	**Endo**	☐ WNL / ☐ Other
Resp	☐ WNL / ☐ Other	**Psych**	☐ WNL / ☐ Other

ROS additional notes

Physical Exam:

Vitals: Pulse: BP: RR: Temp:
SaO_2: Height: Weight: BMI:

General	(NAD, alert, interactive)
HEENT	(NC/AT, MMM, PERRL, EOMI, BL TM intact and reactive to light, BL sclera anicteric)
Neck	(supple, no LAD, no JVD, no thyromegaly)
Cardiovascular	(RRR, S1/S2 normal, no m/r/g)
Respiratory	(CTAB, no r/r/w)
Abdominal	(soft, ND/NT, no masses, normal bowel sounds)
Neurologic	(no focal deficit, CN II-XII intact)
Extremities	(normal tone and ROM)
Skin	(intact, no rashes/lesions/erythema)

Physical exam additional notes:

Labs:

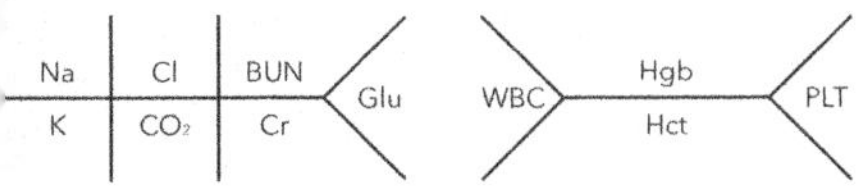

Other Labs:

Studies: (EKG, CXR, other imaging studies)

Impression / Assessment:

Differential Diagnosis:

Plan:

Updates / Notes:

To Do:

Date: Patient Name: Age: Gender:

DOA: Room #: Bed:

Chief Complaint:

History of Present Illness:

Past Medical History: (HTN/DM/CAD/CVA)

Medications:

Past Surgical History:

Family History:

Social History:

Occupation: Lives with: Relationship:

Drug/substance abuse history if any: (alcohol/tobacco/drugs)

Allergies:

Review of Systems: (Describe if not WNL)

General	☐ WNL / ☐ Other	**GI**	☐ WNL / ☐ Other
Skin	☐ WNL / ☐ Other	**GU**	☐ WNL / ☐ Other
ENT	☐ WNL / ☐ Other	**MSK**	☐ WNL / ☐ Other
Eyes	☐ WNL / ☐ Other	**Neuro**	☐ WNL / ☐ Other
CV	☐ WNL / ☐ Other	**Endo**	☐ WNL / ☐ Other
Resp	☐ WNL / ☐ Other	**Psych**	☐ WNL / ☐ Other

ROS additional notes

Physical Exam:

Vitals:	Pulse:	BP:	RR:	Temp:
	SaO_2:	Height:	Weight:	BMI:

General	(NAD, alert, interactive)
HEENT	(NC/AT, MMM, PERRL, EOMI, BL TM intact and reactive to light, BL sclera anicteric)
Neck	(supple, no LAD, no JVD, no thyromegaly)
Cardiovascular	(RRR, S1/S2 normal, no m/r/g)
Respiratory	(CTAB, no r/r/w)
Abdominal	(soft, ND/NT, no masses, normal bowel sounds)
Neurologic	(no focal deficit, CN II-XII intact)
Extremities	(normal tone and ROM)
Skin	(intact, no rashes/lesions/erythema)

Physical exam additional notes:

Labs:

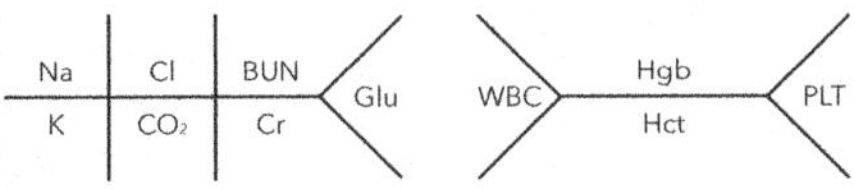

Other Labs:

Studies: (EKG, CXR, other imaging studies)

Impression / Assessment:

Differential Diagnosis:

Plan:

Updates / Notes:

To Do:

Date: Patient Name: Age: Gender:

DOA: Room #: Bed:

Chief Complaint:

History of Present Illness:

Past Medical History: (HTN/DM/CAD/CVA)

Medications:

Past Surgical History:

Family History:

Social History:

Occupation: Lives with: Relationship:

Drug/substance abuse history if any: (alcohol/tobacco/drugs)

Allergies:

Review of Systems: (Describe if not WNL)

General	☐ WNL / ☐ Other	**GI**	☐ WNL / ☐ Other
Skin	☐ WNL / ☐ Other	**GU**	☐ WNL / ☐ Other
ENT	☐ WNL / ☐ Other	**MSK**	☐ WNL / ☐ Other
Eyes	☐ WNL / ☐ Other	**Neuro**	☐ WNL / ☐ Other
CV	☐ WNL / ☐ Other	**Endo**	☐ WNL / ☐ Other
Resp	☐ WNL / ☐ Other	**Psych**	☐ WNL / ☐ Other

ROS additional notes

Physical Exam:

Vitals:	Pulse:	BP:	RR:	Temp:
	SaO_2:	Height:	Weight:	BMI:

General	(NAD, alert, interactive)
HEENT	(NC/AT, MMM, PERRL, EOMI, BL TM intact and reactive to light, BL sclera anicteric)
Neck	(supple, no LAD, no JVD, no thyromegaly)
Cardiovascular	(RRR, S1/S2 normal, no m/r/g)
Respiratory	(CTAB, no r/r/w)
Abdominal	(soft, ND/NT, no masses, normal bowel sounds)
Neurologic	(no focal deficit, CN II-XII intact)
Extremities	(normal tone and ROM)
Skin	(intact, no rashes/lesions/erythema)

Physical exam additional notes:

Labs:

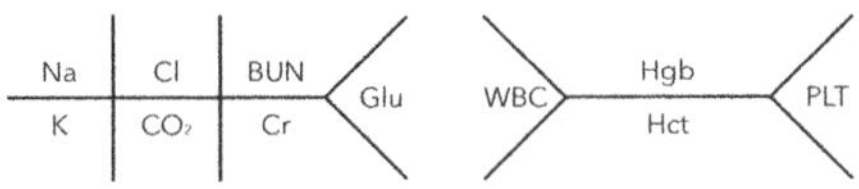

Other Labs:

Studies: (EKG, CXR, other imaging studies)

Impression / Assessment:

Differential Diagnosis:

Plan:

Updates / Notes:

To Do:

Date: Patient Name: Age: Gender:

DOA: Room #: Bed:

Chief Complaint:

History of Present Illness:

Past Medical History: (HTN/DM/CAD/CVA)

Medications:

Past Surgical History:

Family History:

Social History:

Occupation: Lives with: Relationship:

Drug/substance abuse history if any: (alcohol/tobacco/drugs)

Allergies:

Review of Systems: (Describe if not WNL)

General	☐ WNL / ☐ Other	**GI**	☐ WNL / ☐ Other
Skin	☐ WNL / ☐ Other	**GU**	☐ WNL / ☐ Other
ENT	☐ WNL / ☐ Other	**MSK**	☐ WNL / ☐ Other
Eyes	☐ WNL / ☐ Other	**Neuro**	☐ WNL / ☐ Other
CV	☐ WNL / ☐ Other	**Endo**	☐ WNL / ☐ Other
Resp	☐ WNL / ☐ Other	**Psych**	☐ WNL / ☐ Other

ROS additional notes

Physical Exam:

Vitals: Pulse: BP: RR: Temp:
SaO_2: Height: Weight: BMI:

General	(NAD, alert, interactive)
HEENT	(NC/AT, MMM, PERRL, EOMI, BL TM intact and reactive to light, BL sclera anicteric)
Neck	(supple, no LAD, no JVD, no thyromegaly)
Cardiovascular	(RRR, S1/S2 normal, no m/r/g)
Respiratory	(CTAB, no r/r/w)
Abdominal	(soft, ND/NT, no masses, normal bowel sounds)
Neurologic	(no focal deficit, CN II-XII intact)
Extremities	(normal tone and ROM)
Skin	(intact, no rashes/lesions/erythema)

Physical exam additional notes:

Labs:

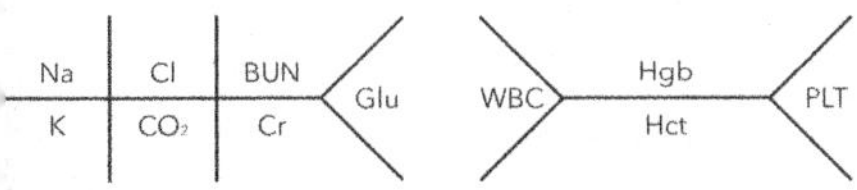

Other Labs:

Studies: (EKG, CXR, other imaging studies)

Impression / Assessment:

Differential Diagnosis:

Plan:

Updates / Notes:

To Do:

Date: Patient Name: Age: Gender:

DOA: Room #: Bed:

Chief Complaint:

History of Present Illness:

Past Medical History: (HTN/DM/CAD/CVA)

Medications:

Past Surgical History:

Family History:

Social History:

Occupation: Lives with: Relationship:

Drug/substance abuse history if any: (alcohol/tobacco/drugs)

Allergies:

Review of Systems: (Describe if not WNL)

General	☐ WNL / ☐ Other	**GI**	☐ WNL / ☐ Other
Skin	☐ WNL / ☐ Other	**GU**	☐ WNL / ☐ Other
ENT	☐ WNL / ☐ Other	**MSK**	☐ WNL / ☐ Other
Eyes	☐ WNL / ☐ Other	**Neuro**	☐ WNL / ☐ Other
CV	☐ WNL / ☐ Other	**Endo**	☐ WNL / ☐ Other
Resp	☐ WNL / ☐ Other	**Psych**	☐ WNL / ☐ Other

ROS additional notes

Physical Exam:

Vitals: Pulse: BP: RR: Temp:
SaO_2: Height: Weight: BMI:

General	(NAD, alert, interactive)
HEENT	(NC/AT, MMM, PERRL, EOMI, BL TM intact and reactive to light, BL sclera anicteric)
Neck	(supple, no LAD, no JVD, no thyromegaly)
Cardiovascular	(RRR, S1/S2 normal, no m/r/g)
Respiratory	(CTAB, no r/r/w)
Abdominal	(soft, ND/NT, no masses, normal bowel sounds)
Neurologic	(no focal deficit, CN II-XII intact)
Extremities	(normal tone and ROM)
Skin	(intact, no rashes/lesions/erythema)

Physical exam additional notes:

Labs:

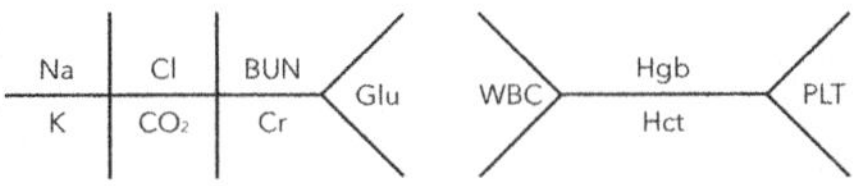

Other Labs:

Studies: (EKG, CXR, other imaging studies)

Impression / Assessment:

Differential Diagnosis:

Plan:

Updates / Notes:

To Do:

Date: Patient Name: Age: Gender:

DOA: Room #: Bed:

Chief Complaint:

History of Present Illness:

Past Medical History: (HTN/DM/CAD/CVA)

Medications:

Past Surgical History:

Family History:

Social History:

Occupation: Lives with: Relationship:

Drug/substance abuse history if any: (alcohol/tobacco/drugs)

Allergies:

Review of Systems: (Describe if not WNL)

General	☐ WNL / ☐ Other	**GI**	☐ WNL / ☐ Other
Skin	☐ WNL / ☐ Other	**GU**	☐ WNL / ☐ Other
ENT	☐ WNL / ☐ Other	**MSK**	☐ WNL / ☐ Other
Eyes	☐ WNL / ☐ Other	**Neuro**	☐ WNL / ☐ Other
CV	☐ WNL / ☐ Other	**Endo**	☐ WNL / ☐ Other
Resp	☐ WNL / ☐ Other	**Psych**	☐ WNL / ☐ Other

ROS additional notes

Physical Exam:

Vitals:	Pulse:	BP:	RR:	Temp:
	SaO_2:	Height:	Weight:	BMI:

General	(NAD, alert, interactive)
HEENT	(NC/AT, MMM, PERRL, EOMI, BL TM intact and reactive to light, BL sclera anicteric)
Neck	(supple, no LAD, no JVD, no thyromegaly)
Cardiovascular	(RRR, S1/S2 normal, no m/r/g)
Respiratory	(CTAB, no r/r/w)
Abdominal	(soft, ND/NT, no masses, normal bowel sounds)
Neurologic	(no focal deficit, CN II-XII intact)
Extremities	(normal tone and ROM)
Skin	(intact, no rashes/lesions/erythema)

Physical exam additional notes:

Labs:

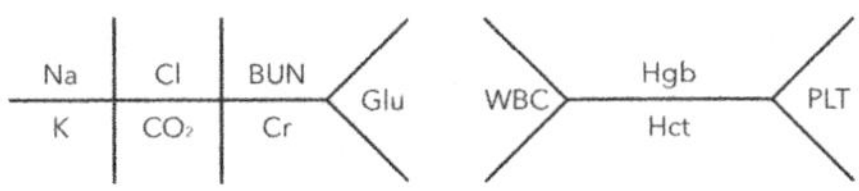

Other Labs:

Studies: (EKG, CXR, other imaging studies)

Impression / Assessment:

Differential Diagnosis:

Plan:

Updates / Notes:

To Do:

Date: Patient Name: Age: Gender:

DOA: Room #: Bed:

Chief Complaint:

History of Present Illness:

Past Medical History: (HTN/DM/CAD/CVA)

Medications:

Past Surgical History:

Family History:

Social History:

Occupation: Lives with: Relationship:

Drug/substance abuse history if any: (alcohol/tobacco/drugs)

Allergies:

Review of Systems: (Describe if not WNL)

General	☐ WNL / ☐ Other	**GI**	☐ WNL / ☐ Other
Skin	☐ WNL / ☐ Other	**GU**	☐ WNL / ☐ Other
ENT	☐ WNL / ☐ Other	**MSK**	☐ WNL / ☐ Other
Eyes	☐ WNL / ☐ Other	**Neuro**	☐ WNL / ☐ Other
CV	☐ WNL / ☐ Other	**Endo**	☐ WNL / ☐ Other
Resp	☐ WNL / ☐ Other	**Psych**	☐ WNL / ☐ Other

ROS additional notes

Physical Exam:

Vitals:	Pulse:	BP:	RR:	Temp:
	SaO_2:	Height:	Weight:	BMI:

General	(NAD, alert, interactive)
HEENT	(NC/AT, MMM, PERRL, EOMI, BL TM intact and reactive to light, BL sclera anicteric)
Neck	(supple, no LAD, no JVD, no thyromegaly)
Cardiovascular	(RRR, S1/S2 normal, no m/r/g)
Respiratory	(CTAB, no r/r/w)
Abdominal	(soft, ND/NT, no masses, normal bowel sounds)
Neurologic	(no focal deficit, CN II-XII intact)
Extremities	(normal tone and ROM)
Skin	(intact, no rashes/lesions/erythema)

Physical exam additional notes:

Labs:

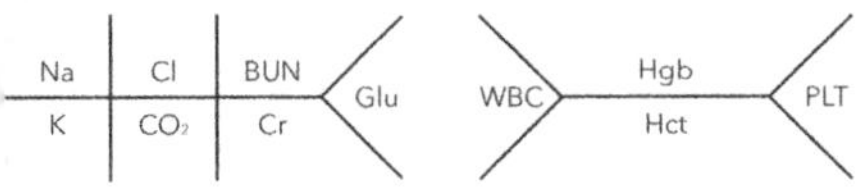

Other Labs:

Studies: (EKG, CXR, other imaging studies)

Impression / Assessment:

Differential Diagnosis:

Plan:

Updates / Notes:

To Do:

Date: Patient Name: Age: Gender:

DOA: Room #: Bed:

Chief Complaint:

History of Present Illness:

Past Medical History: (HTN/DM/CAD/CVA)

Medications:

Past Surgical History:

Family History:

Social History:

Occupation: Lives with: Relationship:

Drug/substance abuse history if any: (alcohol/tobacco/drugs)

Allergies:

Review of Systems: (Describe if not WNL)

General	☐ WNL / ☐ Other	**GI**	☐ WNL / ☐ Other
Skin	☐ WNL / ☐ Other	**GU**	☐ WNL / ☐ Other
ENT	☐ WNL / ☐ Other	**MSK**	☐ WNL / ☐ Other
Eyes	☐ WNL / ☐ Other	**Neuro**	☐ WNL / ☐ Other
CV	☐ WNL / ☐ Other	**Endo**	☐ WNL / ☐ Other
Resp	☐ WNL / ☐ Other	**Psych**	☐ WNL / ☐ Other

ROS additional notes

Physical Exam:

Vitals: Pulse: BP: RR: Temp:
SaO_2: Height: Weight: BMI:

General	(NAD, alert, interactive)
HEENT	(NC/AT, MMM, PERRL, EOMI, BL TM intact and reactive to light, BL sclera anicteric)
Neck	(supple, no LAD, no JVD, no thyromegaly)
Cardiovascular	(RRR, S1/S2 normal, no m/r/g)
Respiratory	(CTAB, no r/r/w)
Abdominal	(soft, ND/NT, no masses, normal bowel sounds)
Neurologic	(no focal deficit, CN II-XII intact)
Extremities	(normal tone and ROM)
Skin	(intact, no rashes/lesions/erythema)

Physical exam additional notes:

Labs:

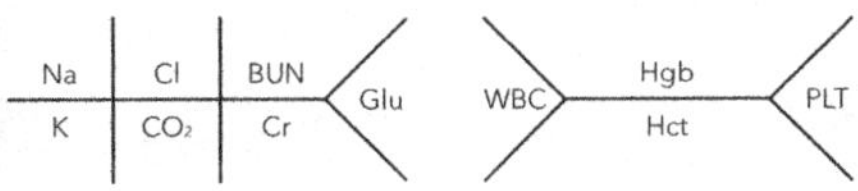

Other Labs:

Studies: (EKG, CXR, other imaging studies)

Impression / Assessment:

Differential Diagnosis:

Plan:

Updates / Notes:

To Do:

LAB VALUES REFERENCE GUIDE

Vitals Pulse: 60-100bpm | BP: 90-120/60-80 mmHg | RR: 12-18 breaths/min
Temp: 97.8 - 99.1°F | SaO_2: 97-100% | BMI: 18.5-24.9

CBC

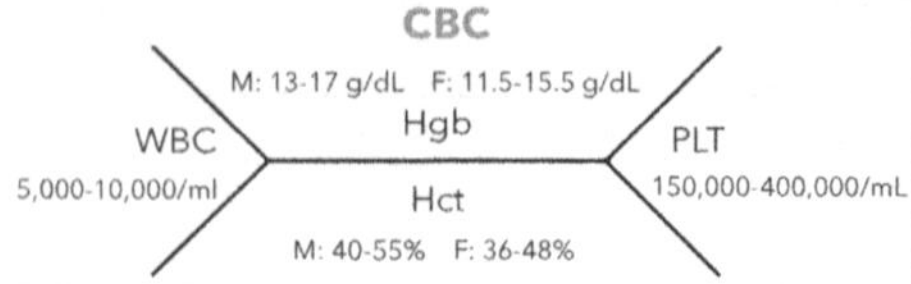

Chem-7

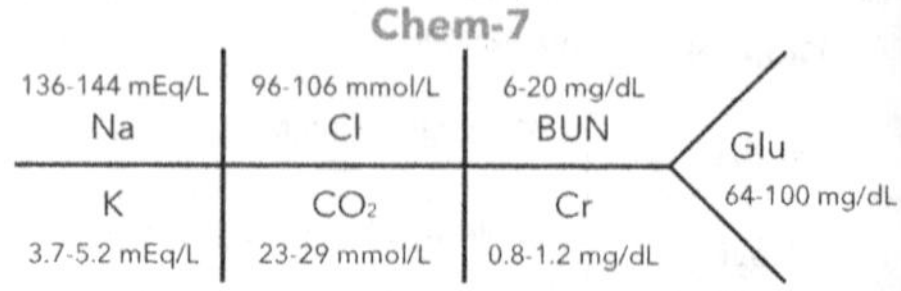

Ca: 8.5-10.5 mg/dl | Mg: 1.7 to 2.2mg/dl
Phosphate: 2.7-4.5 mg/dl

RBC	$4\text{-}6 \times 10^6/\mu L$	Neutrophils	55-73%
MCV	80-100 fl	Bands	0-6%
MCH	26-34 pg	Lymphocytes	20-40%
MCHC	32-36%	Eosinophils	1-4%
ESR	0-20 mm/hr	Monocytes	2-8%
		Basophils	0.5-1%

ABGs

Arterial Blood pH	7.35-7.45
SaO_2	>95%
PCO_2	35-45 mmHg
PaO_2	80-100 mmHg
HCO_3	22-26 mEq/L
Base Excess	±2

Liver Function Tests

Total Bilirubin	0.3-1.0 mg/dL
Direct (conjugated)	0.0-0.2 mg/dL
Indirect (unconjugated)	0.1-1 mg/dL, critical >12
ALT	M: 10-55 units/L
	F: 7-30 units/L
AST	M: 10-40 units/L
	F: 9-25 units/L
ALP	40-130 units/L
Albumin	3.4-5 g/dL
Ammonia	35-65 mcg/dl
Amylase	25-151 units/L
Lipase	10-140 units/L
Protein	6-8 g/dL

Glucose Tests

Glucose, fasting	70-110 mg/dL
Glucose, monitoring	60-110 mg/dL
2-hr Postprandial	<140 mg/dL
HbA1c	7% or lower

Coagulation Tests

APTT	20-60 s
PT	11-13 s, critical >20
Bleeding Time	Duke: 1-3 min
	Ivy: 3-6 min
D-Dimer	<500 ng/mL

Lipoprotein Profile

Cholesterol	<200 mg/dL
HDL	30-70 mg/dL
LDL	<130 mg/dL
Triglycerides	<150 mg/dL

Thyroid Function Tests

T_3	80-230 ng/dL
T_4	5-12 mcg/dL
Free T_4	0.8-2.4 ng/dL
TSH	0.2-5.4 μU/mL

Acid Base Abnormalities

Disorder	pH	HCO_3	$PaCO_2$	Disturbance
Respiratory Acidosis	↓	↑	↑ ↑	Hypoventilation
Respiratory Alkalosis	↑	↓	↓ ↓	Hyperventilation
Metabolic Acidosis	↓	↓ ↓	↓	Loss of HCO_3 or gain of H^+
Metabolic Alkalosis	↑	↑ ↑	↑	Loss of H^+ or gain of HCO_3

Lab Values Reference additional notes: [users can add here any other reference values that they find useful and commonly use in their practice]

CONVERSION GUIDE

Volume	
1 ml	0.034 fluid oz
1 fluid oz	29.6 ml (approx. 30)
1 pint	16 fluid oz
1 pint	473 ml
1 gallon	8 pints
1 gallon	4 quarts
1 liter	1.06 quarts
1 teaspoon	5 ml
1 tablespoon	3 teaspoon

Weight	
1 kg	2.2 pounds (lb)
1 lb	454 g
1 lb	16 ounces (oz)

Temperature	
°F	°C
97.0	36.1
98.6 normal temp	37.0
99.0 fever, armpit	37.2
100.0 fever, oral	37.8
100.4 fever, rectal	38.0
101.0	38.3
°F = (°C × 9/5) + 32	°C = (°F − 32) × 5/9

Length	
1 inch	2.54 cm
1 cm	0.39 inch
1 ft	0.305 m
1 m	3.28 ft

IMPORTANT EQUATIONS

Body Mass Index (BMI)

$$\text{BMI} = \frac{m}{h^2}$$

m: weight in kg; h: height in meters

Cardiac Output (CO)

$$\text{CO} = SV \cdot HR \qquad \frac{ml}{min} = \frac{ml}{beat} \cdot \frac{beat}{min}$$

SV: stroke volume; HR: heart rate

Creatinine Clearance

$$\frac{urine\ creatinine \times urine\ volume}{serum\ creatinine \times time}$$

Anion Gap

$$(\text{AG}) = Na^+ - (Cl^- + HCO_3^-)$$

Body Surface Area

$$BSA(m^2) = \sqrt{\frac{[height(cm) \times weight(kg)}{3600}}$$

Mean Arterial Pressure (mmHg)

$$MAP = DBP + \frac{SBP - DBP}{3}$$

ECG

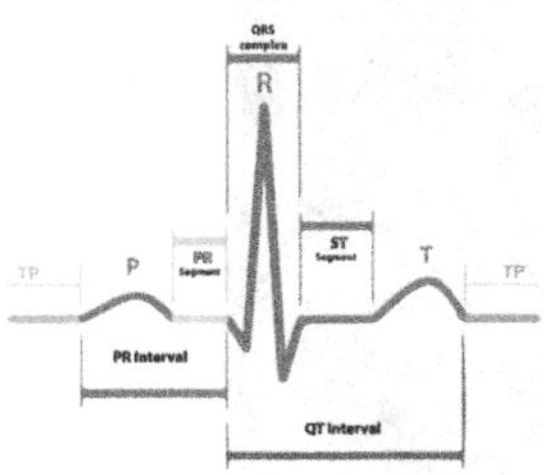

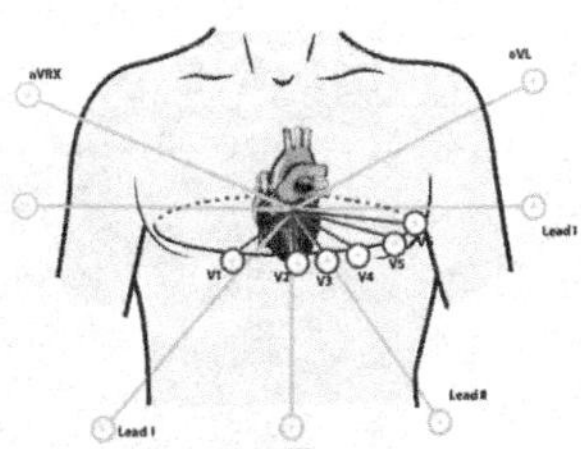

The degree of the QRS axis will tell you whether it is normal or deviated:

- Normal: between -30° to +90°
- Left Axis Deviation (LAD): < -30°
- Right Axis Deviation (RAD): > +90°
- Extreme Axis Deviation (EAD): between -90° & 180°

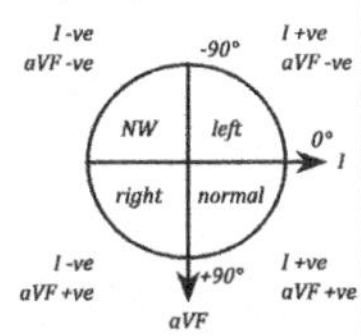

Glasgow Coma Scale (GCS Score)

Eye Opening		Verbal Response		Best Motor Response	
Spontaneous	4	Oriented	5	Obeys commands	6
To sound	3	Confused	4	Localizing to pain	5
To pain	2	Words	3	Normal flexion, withdrawal from pain	4
None	1	Sounds	2	Abnormal flexion, decorticate	3
		None	1	Abnormal extension, decerebrate	2
				None	1

Interpretation:

13-15 = Minor brain injury; 9-12 = Moderate brain injury; 3-8 = Severe brain injury (coma)

Made in the USA
Monee, IL
07 March 2024

54556248R00059